The Healthcare Heist

How Physicians and Patients Can Unite to Transform Healthcare

Jordan Grumet, MD

AAPL

978-1-960762-53-5 print
978-1-960762-54-2 eBook

Published by **American Association for Physician Leadership, Inc.**
PO Box 96503 | BMB 97493 | Washington, DC 20090-6503

Website: www.physicianleaders.org

13 8 7 6 5 4 3 2 1

Copyedited, typeset, indexed, and printed in the United States of America

PUBLISHER
Nancy Collins

PRODUCTION MANAGER
Jennifer Weiss

DESIGN & LAYOUT
Carter Publishing Studio

COPYEDITOR
Patricia George

EARLY PRAISE FOR *The Healthcare Heist: How Physicians and Patients Can Unite to Transform Healthcare*

Patients and doctors are the only ones who really have the ability and the incentive to fix our broken healthcare system. They can no longer neglect their massive power to effect change in the system. Dr. Grumet has defined their opponents in this battle for their money and their very lives. Now it's time for them to use every tool in the arsenal to take back control, including shared storytelling.

Jim and Katie Dahle
THE WHITE COAT INVESTOR

As a veteran ER Physician of "The Pitt," I have seen the once-sacred physician–patient relationship become sadly fractured and transactional. In corporate, "bottom line" medicine and volume-based healthcare, doctors are interchangeable providers and patients are customers on an assembly line. In *The Healthcare Heist*, Dr. Grumet unleashes the power of shared storytelling to restore humanity to healthcare. This book hits Goliath right between the eyes.

Bill Yount, MD
FOUNDER AND COHOST OF THE *CATCHING UP TO FI* PODCAST

As a physician who has served on the literal front lines of combat, I know that true resilience requires trust, unity, and an unwavering commitment to the mission. *The Healthcare Heist* brilliantly exposes how corporate profiteers have intentionally fractured the alliance between doctors and patients, leaving our medical system's foot soldiers defenseless. Dr. Grumet offers a powerful, actionable strategy to rebuild this broken infrastructure and reclaim medicine through shared storytelling and mutual empathy.

Sudip Bose, MD, FACEP, FAAEM
AS SEEN ON *DESERT DOC* ON AMAZON PRIME

This book captures the exact ethos we champion every day on the *KevinMD* blog: the necessity of the physician's voice. Dr. Grumet eloquently proves that when doctors have the courage to share their vulnerability and their struggles, they can inspire a grassroots revolution to save American healthcare.

Kevin Pho, MD
PHYSICIAN AND FOUNDER OF KEVINMD.COM

Jordan Grumet does what the best physician authors do: He uses his own story to tell a much bigger one. *The Healthcare Heist* is part memoir, part indispensable primer on a system that has lost sight of patients, health, and the people delivering care, including doctors. Grumet names the dysfunction and points the reader toward something better.

Resa E. Lewiss, MD
EMERGENCY PHYSICIAN AND HOST OF *THE VISIBLE VOICES* PODCAST

Acknowledgments

WRITING A BOOK IS AN immensely challenging project. After all the blood, sweat and tears, there are many who deserve a hearty thank you for all the time, effort, and guidance they have supplied.

The genesis of this book comes from a talk that I have been privileged to give to medical audiences large and small over the last 10 years. The gift of giving this talk has in most part arisen due to the guidance and friendship of Kevin Pho. He has relentlessly supported my writing and public speaking over the decades and was kind enough to ask me to be part of his speaker's bureau.

To Nancy Collins and the whole staff at the American Association for Physician Leadership. Your organization remains a beacon for those in the trenches of providing our nation's most precious resource — the care we provide for each other.

To Chris Parker who has become a quintessential part of my book writing team. Your input elevates almost every word I place on the page. Your support has been invaluable.

To the many friends who have supported this project and listened to my endless ideas, rants, and complaints: Jason Wojack, JL Collins, Nuno Lieria, Jillian Johnsrud, and Grant Sabatier.

To my mom, dad, and stepdad for your relentless support, knowledge, and upbringing. Most of my good habits were learned long before I knew anything, and came from watching you.

To Katie, Cameron, and Leila. You are my heart and soul. My day and night. My reason for waking up every morning. Thank you for being patient while this book distracted me from your attention. Sometimes I have a one-track mind.

And finally, to all of the patients I have seen over the years and who have allowed me into their struggles. To all the doctors, nurses, chaplains, social workers, therapists, and certified nursing assistants who have given everything to the care of their patients and have often suffered abuse from just about every direction. Our healthcare system couldn't function without you.

Table of Contents

About the Author

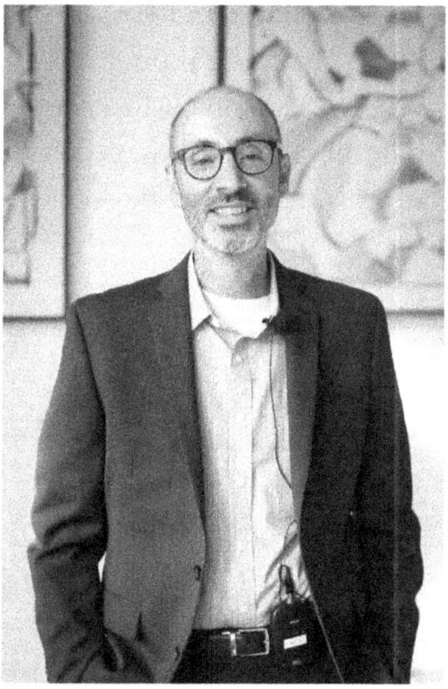

JORDAN GRUMET, BORN IN EVANSTON, ILLINOIS in 1973, found the spark to become a doctor after a deeply personal event reshaped his life's trajectory. The unexpected loss of his father, an oncologist, ignited a passion within him to practice medicine and instilled a unique vantage point that later melded seamlessly with his financial expertise. This convergence of roles has spurred him to explore profound notions like wealth, abundance, and financial independence with a thoughtful and critical lens.

Completing his studies at the University of Michigan, Grumet earned his medical degree from Northwestern University before embarking on a journey in Internal Medicine in Northbrook, Illinois. Presently, he serves as an associate medical director at Unity Hospice.

With a profound understanding of both medicine and finance, Grumet unveiled his thoughts through blogging, specifically focusing on financial independence and wellness. This passion culminated in the launch of the *Earn & Invest* podcast in 2018. His dedication bore fruit in 2019 when he was honored with the Plutus Award for Best New Personal Finance

Podcast, followed by consecutive nominations for Best Personal Finance Podcast of the year in 2020 and 2021.

In August 2022, Grumet's literary pursuit took shape as his book, *Taking Stock: A Hospice Doctor's Advice on Financial Independence, Building Wealth, and Living a Regret-Free Life* was published by Ulysses Press. His second book, *The Purpose Code,* was published January 2025 by Harriman House Press. Jordan's journey intertwines medical insight and financial wisdom, resonating deeply with those seeking a balanced, meaningful life.

Introduction

PNEUMONIA DIDN'T CARE. It wasn't bothered that she was "America's Sweetheart," that she once appeared on the cover of a Wheaties box, nor that she didn't have health insurance. In September 2023, Olympic gold medalist Mary Lou Retton fell ill with a respiratory infection. After a brief hospitalization, she was sent home, but her pneumonia didn't heed the doctor's expectation of a swift recovery. As her breathing progressively worsened, her daughter found her home alone, gasping for air and nearly comatose.

What ensued was a month-long ICU stay in which her loved ones said their last goodbyes and hoped and prayed for a miracle. Retton, as resilient as anyone would expect an Olympian to be, slowly recovered and eventually left the hospital with a weakened body, a portable oxygen tank, and something that she never expected: a huge hospital bill.

Despite a reported net worth as high as $2 million in 2023,[1]Retton simply couldn't afford what many would call a fundamental human right: affordable healthcare. Reflecting on her situation, Retton responded candidly:[2]

> *"When COVID hit and after my divorce and all my pre-existing (conditions), I mean, I've had over 30 operations of orthopedic stuff, I couldn't afford it... But who would even know that this was going to happen to me?"*

While family and friends were relieved that she had not only endured but survived such a traumatic illness, they were faced with the daunting task of paying her medical bills. Eventually, her daughters set up a Go Fund Me page and crowdfunded over $459,000 in donations to cover her care.[3]

Many were critical of Retton's choice not to purchase health insurance. Yet many, too, could identify with her reasons: high deductibles, pre-existing conditions, and a divorce. Situations like Retton's leave us with many important unanswered questions. How do we characterize a country in which beloved athletes and celebrities struggle to secure health insurance in their retirement? Why do even those with substantial wealth find health insurance and medical care cost-prohibitive?

And most critically, how has such desperation arisen in arguably the most wealthy and powerful nation in the world?

Pneumonia didn't care about Mary Lou Retton's lack of health insurance. Why don't we?

WE ARE PAWNS

My medical career ended on an ordinary Wednesday evening with the ring of a doorbell. My family, sitting quietly in the TV room merely feet away, had no idea about the cataclysm that had just overtaken me. When the process server handed me the summons, I felt a brief moment of blissful disconnectedness before I plunged head-first into a dark abyss of burnout, self-doubt, and eventual anger — a rage that would take years to process and even longer to comprehend. From the moment my father died unexpectedly when I was a child — thrusting me toward this career path — I was destined to become an unwitting tool. An instrument. A pawn in a chess match so expansive and all-encompassing that neither I, my patients, nor my fellow caregivers could recognize our roles as merely foot soldiers.

We had become leverage in a lucrative maze of financial and power-based relationships that not only served to drive caregivers and patients apart but threatened to destroy our healthcare system in general.

This realization began for me on that somber winter evening.

Patients as Pawns

I'd be willing to bet that as a patient, you have found our healthcare system to be impersonal and inflexible. You have struggled to receive care, pay for a prescription, or correct inaccuracies in your medical record on a clunky government-mandated patient portal.

The nagging feeling flitted through your brain as you perused your hospital bill, finding that two Tylenol given to you in the emergency room cost your insurance company a staggering $200 each! Or maybe it was the hour and a half spent on hold when trying to get preapproval for a prescription your doctor had repeatedly assured you was vital.

You are challenged by our system even if you are in excellent health. Have you struggled to obtain adequate health insurance after leaving your job and being unable to find inexpensive options on healthcare.gov? When your trusted internist retired at age 45 to pursue a business degree, were you surprised that your new doctor had no availability for at least 10 months?

These scenarios are examples of the not-so-subtle shift in our healthcare system over the past few decades that have created many winners and many losers. The losers in this new world order couldn't be any clearer: It is those who get paid to give care and those who receive that care.

Many of us grew up believing in the inherent fairness and benevolence of our healthcare system. Now, we're left pondering a straightforward question:

If we're not flourishing in this system, who is?

The answer is both glaringly obvious and profoundly painful. Follow the money and the truth emerges. The lone survivors in this dystopian medical landscape are the corporations, venture capitalists, malpractice attorneys, bureaucrats, and other third parties who gain both wealth and power by hijacking our system. They exploit the knowledge and expertise of our healthcare providers and the vulnerability of our patients to squeeze every last penny from our already overburdened medical infrastructure.

It is not too strong to say that these parties are criminally extracting a pound of flesh and providing no tangible return on investment. Many hands dip into the cookie jar — taking often but rarely giving back. Consider this:

- Your health insurance representative doesn't perform your cardiac catheterization.
- Your pharmaceutical company doesn't decide which medications to administer nor titrate the dose.
- Your lawyer doesn't answer the phone late at night when your breathing is tight.
- And the venture capitalist who just bought your primary care physician's practice has no understanding of medical nuance such as the difference between cardiac angina and gastrointestinal dyspepsia.

Yet these are the people responsible for your $200-a-dose of Tylenol. They are responsible for the rigamarole of prior authorizations, duplicate forms, electronic medical records, and *cover-your-ass* charting that pulls doctors and nurses from the bedside in favor of sitting mesmerized in front of computer screens. We are ensnared by a medical system that no longer prioritizes the many but instead is meant to serve the few.

The examples of such behavior are abundant.

Cameron, an 18-year-old unlucky enough to be born with a chronic and debilitating gastrointestinal disease, has discovered first-hand that our healthcare system was not created with his well-being in mind. After struggling for years to eat normally and maintain his body weight, he was prescribed Dupixent, an immunosuppressant that significantly improved his quality of life. Unfortunately, this wonder drug — which costs the pharmaceutical company mere pennies to manufacture — commands a staggering price tag of over $3,000 a dose. While the company justifies these charges with claims of the high cost of research and development, they omit recent data that show **drug manufacturers earn, on average, $18.6 billion in total global revenues for a new drug — 10 times more than the $1.8 billion cost of new drug development.**[4]

"But," you might argue, "that's what healthcare insurance is for."

Yes, Cameron has a fairly generous Blue Cross Blue Shield policy provided by his mother's full-time employer. That employer has agreed to cover the $3,000 for his weekly injections.

That should alleviate most of Cameron's concerns — except that every few months a new prior authorization mysteriously emerges out of thin air, causing delays in shipment and requiring hours of frustrating phone calls to resolve. As a result, Cameron has missed as many doses as he has received, and each missed dose brings about a painful resurgence of symptoms.

Yet his mother diligently pays the premiums and copays, the pharmaceutical company continues posting record profits, and Blue Cross Blue Shield still compensates its chief executive in excess of $22 million a year.[5] If you are naïve enough to believe that the government is here to save Cameron, you, or anyone else from all this chaos, you are sadly mistaken. In reality, our public servants only seem to add to this mess.

Take Lenny, for instance. Since losing his wife to cancer after over 40 years of marriage, he has understandably been suffering from profound depression and anxiety. Attempts to make an appointment with his primary care doctor were initially thwarted by a lack of availability. Eventually, he was offered a slot with a younger colleague, but Lenny hesitated to have such a personal conversation with someone unfamiliar.

After waiting weeks to get an urgent appointment with his preferred doctor, Lenny spent most of the visit watching him type unrelated information into the computer. Despite their decade-long relationship, their time together was marginalized with questions regarding random background and biographical information. The doctor explained that, based on new governmental regulations, he had to populate the chart appropriately.

When, at the very end of the appointment, they were finally able to address Lenny's overwhelming feelings of loss and abandonment, the doctor seemed distracted and hurried to get to his next patient. Lenny was promptly given a referral to see a psychiatrist because the primary care doctor no longer had the time or energy to deal with such "specialized" issues.

There was a catch, though: After dozens of calls, Lenny found that none of the local psychiatrists took health insurance. Exhausted by strikingly low Medicare reimbursement rates and the burden of compliance, many of the doctors in the area had switched to cash-only practices.

And you thought Lenny was depressed before he started his search!

Feeling utterly frustrated and despondent, Lenny eventually turned to the local marijuana dispensary and opted to self-medicate his anxiety. His decision cost him hundreds of dollars out of pocket, tested his time and patience, and saved Medicare (the government) on his psychiatry referral as well as any resulting medication costs.

Providers as Pawns

When you hear politicians tout the low cost of government-run healthcare, now you know why. Accessing care has become so difficult that patients often just give up. Meanwhile, the burden of compliance and administration has been offloaded to hospitals and medical practices. The doctors keep typing on their computers and spend less time than ever actually taking care of patients.

While the suffering of patients and families rightly garners much sympathy, the challenges faced by healthcare providers are often overlooked. Worse yet, third parties perpetuate the divide-and-conquer strategy to mislead people into believing that their doctors are the cause of the systemic problems plaguing our healthcare system.

Physicians have become mere leverage also.

After I endured four years of fear, anxiety, high-priced lawyers' meetings, and eventual depositions, my career-ending malpractice suit — the summons I received on that ordinary Wednesday evening — was thrown out. In the end, the plaintiffs' attorney brazenly admitted that he never believed that I had done anything wrong — he was just hoping to use my testimony as leverage against the nursing home and hospital.

I was being used.

The attorney showed no remorse about how his actions would affect my career, my patients, or even the staff whose jobs depended on my presence and engagement. The patient — whose life expectancy had sadly been measured in days before we met — eventually died because she was elderly, chronically ill, and developed an infection. Even the lawyer realized that trying to sue me, in the end, was futile. But that didn't stop him from finding another party to blame. I had served his purpose as well as his bank account.

Our malpractice system is the poster child for countless other examples in which the doctor-patient relationship is being exploited for profit every day. I remember the sunny spring morning in 2003 when my hospital practice introduced a new electronic medical record system with all its bells and whistles. According to our administrators, it would be the savior of modern-day medicine and patient care. Or, at least, that is what they said as they explained how the burden of populating the system with decades of medical history and biographical information would fall squarely on doctors' and nurses' shoulders without any extra compensation.

We sacrificed our time and energy, redirecting attention away from patient care to appease our new digital overlords. Years later, after billions of dollars have lined the pockets of electronic medical records companies and countless advances have been made to help hospitals and medical centers use them to bill even more for medical care, medical outcomes are no better. Medical errors are no fewer.

Care is slower, less organized, and less available than ever. And the electronic medical records companies are filling their accounts with money that was originally earmarked to improve patient care.

MAY I HAVE THIS DANCE?

Many individuals, like Cameron and Lenny, are struggling to navigate through our healthcare system at this very moment. Many healthcare providers are burdened by the threat of malpractice or the overregulation spurred by our own government and insurers. Yet we often turn to the very entities responsible for our current problems to provide solutions.

Consider the trend toward privatization of healthcare. Medicare Advantage — private company-offered health plans that are a market-based alternative — has encroached on traditional Medicare. Not-for-profit healthcare systems are being outcompeted by private equity or audited into submission, increasing the pressure to sell to for-profit entities. These entities, seeing the distress of the not-for-profits as a ripe opportunity for growth at a low cost, are buying up medical practices, extended care facilities, and hospital systems at a rapid rate.[6] And that's alarming for anyone who prioritizes health access and outcomes over short-term profits.

We are letting the foxes loose in the hen house and the American public is starting to look a lot like hens.

The consequences are profound: not only are our citizens facing financial ruin and the degradation of our once-superior healthcare system, but also a rending of the fabric of the doctor (or healthcare-giver) and patient relationship. This trajectory traces its roots back to 1999 with the publication of the sentinel report from the institute of medicine titled *To Err is Human*, which claimed that medical errors accounted for 44,000 to 98,000 deaths per year in American hospitals.[7]

While these figures and the extent of the harm they represent have been much debated, the conclusions have inflicted lasting damage. The image of doctors created by such reports was that of lazy, rich, fat cats indifferent to patient safety. Many people were led to believe that patients were dying in hospitals on a regular basis and physicians were doing nothing about it; even worse, they were causing the deaths themselves.

Adding to this narrative over the last two decades was the tidal wave of healthcare "reform" that reinforced the role of doctors as the holders of the purse strings. The rise of HMOs and the gatekeeper model that started in the 1980s, and more recently accountable care organizations, places the responsibility squarely on physicians' shoulders to deny care.

Doctors became viewed by the greater public not only as indifferent and careless, but also needlessly frugal with our nation's healthcare resources.

Meanwhile the Centers for Medicare & Medicaid Services (CMS) began to squeeze physicians in an entirely different direction. They enlisted Medicare administrative contractors — third-party businesses to oversee physician compliance with coding and billing regulations — and increased the number of audits to root out much ballyhooed "fraudulent" physicians. While "education audits" sound not only innocuous but also possibly beneficial, these third-party entities are incentivized to recover funds from physicians and hospitals, creating all sorts of conflicts of interest. The more they claw back, the more they get paid.

Is it a wonder that, without fail, every audited physician and hospital is eventually found to be in violation?

Doctors and nurses bogged down with overcompliance, overregulation, and the dictates of the electronic medical record system find that time carries a steep premium. Less time is spent face-to-face with patients and more is dedicated to administrative tasks behind computer screens. Even when we are in the exam room, we are distracted by the overwhelming necessity of data collection.

This distractedness widens the gap between harried healthcare practitioners and an already-skeptical populace. We make less eye contact. We shake fewer hands. We certainly don't hug our patients anymore.

Doctors and patients have been weaponized against each other. We find ourselves sitting on opposite sides of the jury. On opposite sides of the computer screen. And often caught in the middle of an awkward dance with insurance companies, the pharmaceutical industry, and the government. Our waltz is to provide or receive the best possible care. Their tango is to make a fortune at our expense.

These dances are anything but harmonious and we are finding our hands and feet in all the wrong places. We are no longer moving in-step.

I would love to pretend that the lines of battle have been drawn innocently and that the confrontational postures of doctors and patients have arisen organically and without malice. But that would be a huge mistake.

As doctors and patients point fingers at each other, third parties are tiptoeing into the bank vault and emptying our safety deposit boxes of all of our valuables. If they can just keep us distracted long enough — angry enough at each other — maybe no one will notice that we are being robbed blind.

Our very existence depends on seeing through this deception. Our access to life-saving healthcare hangs in the balance.

The aim of this book is to highlight the erosion of the doctor–patient relationship and give examples of how third parties exploit doctors and patients to fulfill their own needs. We must aggressively scrutinize how the commercialization and regulation of healthcare is destroying the lives of those in need. Yet I would be negligent if I didn't pose any remedies to the variety of problems that plague us.

Let me start by conceding that I have no specific laws to suggest, legislation to support, nor political agenda to propose. We are long past the point where such recommendations alone could halt the runaway train that is our healthcare system. Instead, I offer a far bolder and sweeping alternative. We don't need to just change healthcare — we need to revolutionize it.

YOU SAY YOU WANT A REVOLUTION

To fix our healthcare system, we must fundamentally rewrite the rules of engagement. As with any revolution, we must unite the major stakeholders with the bonds of allyship. Only then will we garner a consensus robust enough to turn the tide of third-party greed and manipulation.

When I speak of stakeholders, I am referring to the only two groups that truly matter in any healthy system: (1) those who deliver care and (2) those in need of care.

That's it. Healthcare providers and patients. Those with the expertise and those requiring it.

All other parties are extraneous: hospital boards, administrators, insurance firms, pharmaceutical executives, malpractice attorneys, electronic medical record providers, pharmaceutical representatives — anyone who profits from our healthcare system without directly delivering care to those in need.

The more challenging task is to determine how to unite these stakeholders in order to begin the process of initiating the grass roots change that will ignite a revolution. How do we mend that which has been fractured?

My solution is straightforward yet powerful: **Use shared storytelling as a means to overcome the intimacy gap**.

DEFINING THE INTIMACY GAP

What is the intimacy gap?

I used to believe there was a communication gulf between doctors and patients. Somewhere in the hubbub of the harried office visit some secret sauce was missing. It was a divide so profound that often both parties left the exam room feeling disjointed and uneasy. Patients felt like no one was listening to their complaints. Doctors felt that no one was heeding their advice. The tension ebbed and flowed but never went away completely.

I have since come to realize that the term "communication" is inadequate. It lacks specificity. What we really have is an intimacy gap. What separates doctors from patients is a disjointed and unnatural version of intimacy that in no way reflects the important bonds that form in real-life non-medical relationships.

Let me explain. A patient walks into the office and unloads the most intimate and embarrassing secrets. Unlike the patient's family or friends, the doctor has in no way earned the privilege of hearing these intimate secrets. The doctor hasn't gained the right through hours of conversation, years of support, or selfless acts. There is no shared struggle or trust. The information is given too easily.

The doctor listens patiently, kindly. But the interaction can only be so rewarding. There is no bidirectional flow of intimacy. No mutual disclosure of secrets. The doctor listens without emotion. This is what doctors are taught in our clinical training: disjointed, unnatural intimacy.

So far, we as a society have not solved this problem. For my part, I have decided to strive for mutual disclosure. Maybe we as doctors need to tell our stories to those we care for.

It is through the sharing of these stories that barriers dissolve and we become not doctor and patient, nor teacher and student, but equals. It is in this equality that we will discover redemption and cultivate the political will to rid ourselves of overly interested third parties who see the health of America as a perpetual revenue stream.

It is in this equality that revolution will ultimately take root.

I can sense your skepticism as you read these words. I grappled with the same doubts at the onset of my medical practice in the early 2000s. The notion of sharing my stories with non-medical people seemed absurd.

Yet I forged ahead anyway. I began a blog called *In My Humble Opinion* in which I candidly depicted life on the other side of the stethoscope. The stories I told were full of joy and hope as well as sadness and sorrow. My pain and awe were expressed in equal parts. My blood was on the page available for all to see.

As the years passed and more and more patients read my reflections, I began to realize that the responses were almost always the same: *"I had no idea my doctor felt such things, experienced such things."*

They hadn't realized that my anxious demeanor or terse responses on any given Tuesday weren't about them but were more reflective of the devastating news that I had just delivered to the young couple who huddled in the next room crying. They weren't aware of the late-night phone call the previous night, nor that my favorite patient had just died in the ICU of the local hospital. They didn't know of the countless stressors, worries, and nail-biting moments that make up the average doctor's day in the office. They didn't know **because no one had shared these stories with them**.

It is time we told our stories. Time we shattered the protective barriers that have not only shielded the public from our realities but also locked in the trauma that has ravaged our psyches. We must replace walls with bridges.

BUILDING BRIDGES

This book is my bridge to you. I am extending my hands and asking you to join me. Within these pages you will read stories of how caregivers and patients have been exploited by a system that has been created to serve others' priorities. We will examine the pharmaceutical and insurance industries and uncover their motives, including but not limited to record profits. We will place a magnifying glass on governmental overregulation, failed bureaucracy, and how venture capital and private equity have stepped in to fill the void. We will place a spotlight on how our system of malpractice in the United States serves lawyers more than victims of poor medical judgement. And finally, I will show how true and enduring change in our medical systems has historically and will continue to come from shared storytelling.

This is the beginning of a revolution!

My goal is to help you see that the artificial separation between doctors and patients, caregivers and the cared for, is unnecessary, and has been created to exploit the system.

Lastly, I will share with you some of the stories of the men and women who have dedicated their lives to helping their fellow human beings. We will discuss their struggles and triumphs. Not to celebrate them. Not to laud them as any higher or lower than the patients they serve. But, instead, to create intimacy.

These are our stories. This is our humanity.

Let's fix our healthcare system.

PART ONE.

When Patients Become Customers

IN 1951, A YOUNG MOTHER OF FIVE named Henrietta Lacks sought treatment at Johns Hopkins University Hospital for a complaint of vaginal bleeding.[1] During her physical exam, doctors found a large tumor on her cervix and a biopsy was sent to the laboratory. This tissue, eventually known as HeLa cells, was collected by Dr. George Gey in the laboratory and cultured.

To Dr. Gey's astonishment, instead of dividing a few times and dying, the cells began doubling almost every 24 hours. Despite Mrs. Lacks passing later that year at the age of 31, her cells were grown in the laboratory and eventually used for an array of medical purposes including research, development of therapeutics, and even COVID vaccines, all without her or her family's knowledge or consent.

More than 70 years after Henrietta Lacks' tissue was taken and used without her permission, her descendants reached a settlement with a biotechnology company that they claimed reaped billions of dollars from using her biologic material.[2] According to the lawsuit: "Thermo Fisher Scientific has known that HeLa cells were stolen from Ms. Lacks and chose to use her body for profit anyway."[3]

In the first part of this book, we explore how third parties continue to use our bodies for profit. Instead of our cells, however, they are capitalizing on our dire need for medical services. We have ceased to be treated as patients and have been reduced to nothing more than customers.

First, some history: Who is the U.S. healthcare system meant to serve? Reflecting on our history as a country reveals a time when routine medical care was often provided for the community by the community. In colonial times, with fewer upper-class physicians making the journey to the new world, women colonists often took on the role of caring for the pregnant and the chronically ill.[4] Government regulation was minimal, and it wasn't until 1765 that the first medical college was established in Philadelphia.

The 1800s brought the Civil War, which ushered in advances in surgical techniques, nursing methods, and the care of the acutely ill, all for the benefit of the troops and eventually everyday civilians. Post-war, in 1886, the U.S. army established the Hospital Corps and eventually the Library of the Surgeon General's Office.[4]

The rise of private insurance, both not-for-profit as well as for-profit, coincided with the industrial revolution and the formation of unions seeking to offset financial losses due to injury and illness.[4] This trend accelerated with World War II when businesses, constrained by wartime salary caps, began offering employer-sponsored healthcare to retain valuable employees. These businesses contracted with newly minted health insurers like Blue Cross to provide hospital services and Blue Shield to pay for physician care.[5]

The U.S. pharmaceutical industry started with a similar focus on public welfare. Companies like Pfizer in the north and Eli Lilly in the south originated as efforts to provide lifesaving anesthetics and pain medicines during the Civil War.[6]

Fast forward to the 1950s and the U.S. pharmaceutical industry was experiencing rapid expansion. According to PharmPhorum.com:[6]

> *"The U.S. pharmaceutical industry was booming, thanks to being part of the world's biggest and most dynamic economy. Its growth was also helped by generous funding from the government, with the National Institutes of Health seeing its federal funding rise to nearly $100 million by 1956. This investment fueled the development of drugs to come over the coming decades."*

With this growth, a shift began. While public health undoubtedly benefited from the development of drugs, so did an industry — and with that came other incentives and forces. It was the start of transition away from a focus on public health and toward the medical sector becoming a lucrative profit center. It was the beginning of the commoditization of caregiving.

Instead of simply being patients, individuals seeking medical care were increasingly viewed by an ever-growing cohort of healthcare entrepreneurs as customers who needed to be marketed to, confused, and eventually duped in the name of the almighty dollar. Part one of this book will detail the consequences of this transformation, highlighting how it has led to outsized financial windfalls for Big Pharma, Big Insurance, and Big Business, while deliberately undermining the doctor-patient relationship.

And how we all lose because of it.

CHAPTER ONE.

Is Your Doctor Your Frenemy? (The Patient's View)

WHILE DR. WEISS HAD ALWAYS BEEN KIND in person, Lana's patience was starting to wear thin. After years of struggling to find the right blood pressure pill, they finally settled on carvedilol. It not only brought her systolic blood pressure down nicely, but for once Lana had no side effects — no dizziness, nausea, abdominal pain, or even constipation.

Lana's relief, however, quickly turned to frustration. At first, it was the pharmacy. According to the technician, Dr. Weiss hadn't "bothered" to call in the prescription. But Lana knew that was not the truth — she saw her electronically send the script from the computer in the exam room.

Perplexed, she called her insurer to investigate what was causing the holdup. According to the operator at the call center, carvedilol was no longer covered on the insurer's formulary. After Lana spent an hour explaining that this was the only medicine that worked, the operator acknowledged that Dr. Weiss had indeed submitted the prescription but had not yet responded to the prior-authorization request from the health insurance company.

Fuming and feeling like she had already wasted too much time, Lana was on the verge of giving Dr. Weiss's secretary a piece of her mind when the truth ultimately emerged. Dr. Weiss herself had been on hold for 45 minutes that morning trying to get the prior authorization approved. However, when an urgent situation arose in the emergency room, she rushed out of the office and had to hang up the phone before speaking to a live person.

And finally, after much aggravation and when all seemed lost, the pharmacy called later that day to let Lana know that her prescription was ready. Despite all the hassle, the insurance formulary hadn't yet been updated and carvedilol was actually covered.

WHEN ALL ELSE FAILS, BLAME THE DOCTOR

Lana's experience is far from uncommon. There are countless Dr. Weisses out there unfairly shouldering the blame for just about all the systemic issues that plague our healthcare system. Dr. Brian Johnston articulated this well in his 2021 letter to the editor of the *LA Times* titled, "This is why blaming doctors is pointless: America has no healthcare system":[1]

> *"Our insurance companies take the premiums as profit and avoid their fiduciary duty to pay for the services rendered. Our pharmaceutical industry has gouged the American public while creating an opioid epidemic. Healthcare industry executives have garnered exorbitant compensation while shortchanging patients and those providing the care.*
>
> *We have spent decades debating whether healthcare is a right or a privilege, while never acknowledging that healthcare is a universal necessity. Our healthcare problems do not begin or end with doctors, nurses or any individual group. They begin where we deny that healthcare is a common good."*

A significant part of the problem lies in seeing healthcare as anything less than a common good and, therefore, allowing third parties to game the system in search of higher profits. Unlike buying cars or televisions, if we receive cheap medical treatment, we can't just follow some return policy or trade up for a better model. The consequences are often devastating and irreversible. The result is a divide-and-conquer strategy that pits doctors and patients against each other in order to better serve a number of profiteers including health insurers, Big Pharma, and the American medicolegal complex.

Let's briefly consider how these third parties villainize physicians in the eyes of patients.

BIG INSURANCE MEANS BIG MONEY

Health insurers have long touted their role in shielding patients from exorbitant costs and healthcare liabilities. However, as exposed in a 2018 NPR/*ProPublica* article titled "Why Your Health Insurer Doesn't Care

About Your Big Bills," these claims often conceal a harsh reality.[2] The deception typically begins with routine medical needs like an elective hip replacement. Insurers negotiate an initial in-network fee — such as the $70,882 cited in the article. Patients are then responsible for a 10% coinsurance directly to the hospital ($7,088). Yet, the insurer has little motivation to drive down the original price closer to Medicare rates, which can be as low as a third of the negotiated price. Instead, they offset the rising cost of claims by increasing premiums annually. This lack of downward price pressure persists because insurers can easily price in the increase in overhead costs and adjust premiums accordingly, adding a 20% buffer for administrative fees. In some cases, insured patients end up paying more out-of-pocket than those without insurance coverage.

A 2021 *New York Times* article highlights the irony of federal regulations meant to cap insurers' profits as a percentage of total care expenditures.[3] Paradoxically, these regulations incentivize insurers to maximize payouts, as each dollar spent on care potentially increases their profits as long as they simply charge higher premiums. The cycle perpetuates itself, enabling insurers to profit regardless of their effectiveness in controlling healthcare costs.

While experts often point fingers at doctors in regard to high prices, the reality is that much of the blame falls on for-profit hospitals that, for obvious reasons, are incentivized to inflate prices and then pass on the costs to insurers. Consequently, patients are stuck paying higher premiums, higher copays and coinsurance, and larger deductibles.

If you suspect that physicians are profiting excessively from this plundering of American's bank accounts, you would be sadly mistaken. The majority of physicians, in fact, are transitioning from employers and owners of private practices to mere employees. According to the American Medical Association,[4] 2020 marked the first year in which more than 50% of practicing physicians were employed rather than owning their practices.

The shift is driven by the escalating cost of delivering healthcare in general, including higher practice overhead, increased governmental and insurer compliance and regulation, a rising cost of technology, and fierce competition from larger for-profit entities that operate on economies of scale and treat primary care as a loss leader.

Ultimately it seems insurers, surgical centers, and hospitals end up the winners. Patients and doctors are left to suffer the consequences. Yet we don't acknowledge our shared predicament.

BIG PHARMA, BIG DRAMA

There is no denying that there is an enormous ethical grey area in the relationship between physicians and pharmaceutical companies. To assert otherwise would be laughable given that some doctors receive "consulting" fees that reach into the seven figures. According to *ProPublica,* in a five-year period, 2,500 doctors received at least $500,000 in payments, with 700 surpassing $1 million in total.[5] Considering that there are more than 1.5 million doctors (the numbers in their investigation included dentists, chiropractors, and other healthcare practitioners — not just MDs), the data are slightly less remarkable. It is also important to note that many of these doctors are full-time consultants or speakers, and thus their face time with patients is limited.

ProPublica further reported 1 million doctors, dentists, optometrists, chiropractors, and podiatrists received at least one "payment," most often a meal, from a pharmaceutical company. Various organizations have analyzed payment data in relation to prescribing practices and concluded that these "contributions" indeed do benefit the promotion and sales of specific drugs.

In fact, to address this issue, the government introduced section 6002 of the Affordable Care Act, known as the Physician Payments Sunshine Act. This legislation requires medical product manufacturers to publicly disclose payments made to physicians and teaching hospitals. Interestingly, of the three entities targeted (doctors, hospitals, and pharma) only physicians were explicitly named in the Act's title — a fact not lost on many clinicians.

It's worth mentioning that these investigations often overlook the fact that while the majority of physicians earn modestly little from these relationships in comparison to their wages from doctoring, pharmaceutical companies allocate more on marketing than they do on research and development. Table 1 speaks volumes. The noted disparity underscores the fiduciary responsibility of these companies to market by whatever legal means available to them.

Pharmaceutical Company Spending on Marketing vs. Research & Development in 2019

Pharmaceutical Company	2019 Annual Revenue (in millions)	Money (in millions) Spent on Research & Development	Money (in millions) Spent on Marketing and Sales
Eli Lilly	$22,320	$5,595	$6,204
GlaxoSmithKline	€21,891	€4,568	€11,402
Pfizer	$51,750	$8,650	$14,350
Novartis	$34,252	$9,402	$14,369
AbbVie	$33,266	$6,942	$7,439

PharmacyChecker Research July 2020

TABLE 1. Pharmaceutical Company Spending on Marketing vs. Research and Development

Less frequently discussed, however, is the systemic and often under-publicized grooming of medical students, residents, and young doctors by Big Pharma. As highlighted by Rijul Kshirsager and Priscilla Vu at *in-Training* a medical student community site:[6]

> *"Medical students are subjected to a barrage of advertising that inevitably leads to a physician-industry connection that can be harmful to our health care system. Medical students' exposure to pharmaceutical marketing begins early, growing in frequency throughout their training. Students receive gifts such as free meals, textbooks, pocket texts, small trinkets and even drug samples. Pharmaceutical companies, recognizing the formative nature of the clinical years of medical education, seek to form relationships with medical students years before they are ready to independently practice medicine.*
>
> *"These interactions intensify throughout a physician's training, ranging from trivial gifts such as pens and pads to more questionable large honoraria and consulting fees.*

"As medical students are increasingly subjected to pharmaceutical marketing throughout their education, their skepticism towards the practices of the pharmaceutical industry gradually diminishes. In losing their ability to detect bias and analyze pharmaceutical marketing statements objectively, medical students hinder their future ability to practice evidence-based medicine."

This grooming process creates an unholy alliance that, admittedly, benefits both parties. However, it is important to note that the monetary benefits to most physicians, in the long run, are meager compared to the substantial profits reaped by pharmaceutical companies. For example, a 2017 study in the *Journal of General Internal Medicine* revealed that while 65% of patients studied saw a doctor who received payments, the median amount when compared to overall income was laughably small: just $510.[7]

While doctors are not exempt from public scrutiny, their role in extracting wealth from the American people pales in comparison to the pharma industry's scale. Maybe the legislation should be renamed to reflect this reality: The Pharmaceutical Industry Fleecing of America Sunshine Act!

Speaking of fleecing, it is worth noting the role malpractice lawyers play in the destruction of our healthcare system. While Chapter Six delves deeply into the American medicolegal complex, revealing how it effectively channels wealth from citizens to lawyers, it is important here to note that trust has eroded and blame has been firmly placed. As Chapter Six will elaborate, the narrative that lawyers are here to protect us from incompetent doctors is harmful and yet persists nonetheless.

ARE DOCTORS OVERPAID?

Arguably one of the most damaging assertions driving a wedge between doctors and patients revolves around money. In fact, the tiresome trope that greedy American doctors are responsible for the decline of our healthcare system has been relentlessly voiced in the media. For instance, Dean Baker, co-director of the Center for Economic and Policy Research, a progressive think tank focused on economic policy, succinctly stated this viewpoint in a 2017 *Politico* opinion piece:[8]

"But if we want to stop paying a $100 billion premium for health care that doesn't make us healthier, we're going to need to overcome

> *those political barriers. Getting U.S. health care costs down is a herculean task; getting doctors' pay in line is a big part of the solution. It's time we broke up the doctor cartel."*

While comparing the medical profession to a cartel is hardly beneficial, I can appreciate his perspective. Let's compare the United States to other countries. Medscape's 2024 Physician Compensation report noted that the average annual income for American physicians is $363,000 per year.[9] Diving deeper, specialists earn an average of $394,000 per year while primary care physicians average $277,000 annually. This places physicians among the top 2%–5% of all income earners in the United States. In contrast, our counterparts in countries like Canada earn around $255,000 per year in American dollars, and in the UK, the average is approximately $115,000. These disparities are undeniable.

Furthermore, Dean Baker highlights how physician shortages and the resultant increase in salaries may have been intentionally created. While there is no shortage of young people who want to become doctors, or even foreign-born and trained medical graduates eager to join the American system, the bottleneck lies in the limited number of residency spots available due to Medicare's graduate medical funding, which has been capped by legislation since 1997. Although recent changes have attempted to remedy the situation, these constraints have severely limited our nation's capacity to train new physicians.

Baker rightly points out that some of these funding restrictions were influenced by lobbying efforts from physician advocacy groups. Notably, the American Medical Association, which has generally opposed funding increases, has, since 2019, been calling for an increase in the size and number of medical schools along with the creation of more than 15,000 new residency slots.[10] The AMA defends this about-face by noting that the number of physicians has quadrupled since 1965, far outpacing population growth.

Thus, the larger question remains whether physicians are just highly compensated or indeed overpaid. Moreover, would fixing the perceived situation actually move the needle on overall healthcare costs? In the following sections, we will delve into these questions and explore a few related topics to provide a broader perspective.

The Cost of a Good Education and the Loss of Opportunity

Let's begin with the cost of pursuing a medical education in America. As of 2022, the average annual cost of medical school in the United States was $55,000, with some institutions charging up to $70,000 per year.[11] This results in the average medical student graduating with a staggering $242,000 of debt, with some accruing as much as $400,000 in loans. Contrast this to Canadian students who spend slightly less than $17,000 annually on medical education.[12]

Now let's consider the opportunity cost of attending medical school. Generally, medical training in the United States requires four years of undergraduate college, followed by four years of medical school, and then residency, which can range from three to seven years. This timeline excludes fellowship training, which can add an additional one to three years. Thus, it could take anywhere from a minimum of 11 to a maximum of 18 years to become a practicing physician. Importantly, the first eight years of this journey are entirely uncompensated and come with significant economic sacrifices.

During residency and fellowship, doctors are finally compensated, but their salary remains relatively low. According to Medscape's 2022 Resident Salary and Debt report, the average take-home pay for residents was $64,000 annually, despite typically working 60 to 80 hours a week.[13] This translates to an hourly wage of approximately $21 based on a 60-hour work week.

While physicians' income increases substantially after completing their training, this often occurs when they are well into their 30s, having spent more than a decade accumulating compounded undergraduate and medical school debt. Meanwhile, their peers have had nearly a decade head start when it comes to working and saving — a process they potentially began in their early 20s.

In summary, the path to becoming a physician in the United States starts with substantial financial burdens and entails significant delayed gratification, placing aspiring doctors squarely behind the eight ball.

Are Doctors the Only Ones Being Overpaid in Healthcare?

If we propose that American physicians are being overpaid, then the natural follow-up question is: *in comparison to whom*? Considering the extensive years of training, technical expertise, and necessary experience to provide medical care, who else in the healthcare arena would be a suitable comparison?

Could healthcare executives and administrators be a relevant comparator? According to the AFL-CIO's annual executive compensation report, CEOs received substantial compensation in 2020 with figures reaching up to as much as $15.5 million.[14] For instance, Samuel Hazen, CEO of Nashville-based HCA Healthcare, received $30.4 million, and Ronald Rittenmayer, CEO of Tenet Healthcare, received a reported $16.7 million. I suspect neither of them underwent seven or more years of post-graduate training nor made daily decisions that held people's lives directly in their hands.

Individual hospital CEOs typically earn between $274,000 and $1 million per year, depending on the size of their hospital's revenues. In fact, a 2018 study published in *Clinical Orthopedics and Related Research* concludes:[15]

> *"There is a fast-rising wage gap between the top executives of major nonprofit centers and physicians that reflects the substantial, and growing, cost of nonclinical worker wages to the US healthcare system. However, there does not appear to be a proportionate increase in healthcare utilization. These findings suggest a growing, substantial burden of nonclinical tasks in healthcare."*

The disparities become even more pronounced when we examine how pharmaceutical companies pay their CEOs. Details from a 2023 report from the Senate Committee on Health, Education, Labor, & Pensions[16] reveals some staggering figures.

Table 2 clearly illustrates that CEOs and top executives not only received millions of dollars in salary and benefits, but were also *gifted* lucrative golden parachutes upon their departure.

And the bounty is not just limited to pharmaceutical companies. According to *STAT*, the seven highest-paid health insurance CEOs collectively earned upwards of a whopping $283 million in 2021 alone.[17] Clearly, being part of the healthcare industry is quite economically rewarding, but it appears that physicians, in particular, are severely undervalued. While

COMPANY[21]	2021 CEO COMPENSATION AND GOLDEN PARACHUTES	2021 TOP EXECUTIVES' TOTAL COMPENSATION
abbvie	**President Richard A. Gonzalez** made nearly **$62 million** and could receive more than **$113 million** when he leaves the company	Top five executives took home over **$140 million** in compensation
AMGEN	**CEO Robert A. Bradway** made more than **$48 million** in compensation and could receive more than **$36 million** when he leaves the company	Top five executives took home over **$92 million** in compensation and stock awards
Bristol Myers Squibb	**CEO Giovanni Caforio** made more than **$33 million** and could receive more than **$37 million** when he leaves the company	Top five executives took home **$85 million** in compensation and stock awards
Lilly	**President & CEO David A. Ricks** made more than **$67 million** in compensation and could receive over **$91 million** when he leaves the company	Top five executives took home over **$104 million** in compensation and stock awards
GILEAD	**CEO Daniel P. O'Day** made more than **$23 million** in compensation and could receive nearly **$61 million** when he leaves the company	Top five executives took home nearly **$52 million** in compensation
Johnson & Johnson	**Chairman & CEO Alex Gorsky** made more than **$39 million** in compensation and could receive over **$56 million** when he leaves the company	Top five executives took home more than **$103 million** in compensation
MERCK	**CEO Robert M. Davis** made more than **$17 million** In compensation and could receive nearly **$22 million** when he leaves the company	Top five executives took home more than **$107 million** in compensation and stock awards
moderna	**CEO Stéphane Bancel** made over **$18 million** in compensation and could receive more than **$926 million** when he leaves the company	Top five executives took home over **$409 million** in compensation and stock awards
REGENERON	**CEO Leonard S. Schleifer** made nearly **$453 million** In compensation and could receive almost **$130 million** when he leaves the company	Top five executives took home nearly **$718 million** in compensation and stock awards
Pfizer	**Chairman & CEO Albert Bourla** made more than **$31 million** and could receive nearly **$113 million** when he leaves the company	Top five executives took home more than **$86 million** in compensation

TABLE 2. Pharmaceutical Executive Compensation Trends in 2021.[16]

one could debate the comparability of a rank-and-file physician to that of a pharmaceutical CEO, is the discrepancy truly justified by a factor of 100?

I'm having trouble seeing the problem with physician salaries.

American White-Collar Workers Are Just Paid Well in Some Sectors

In reality, American workers are generously compensated in many sectors, and the disparities are even more pronounced than is the case with physicians. For instance, Qubit conducted research on average salaries from software engineers across the globe utilizing salary calculators such as SalaryExpert, Glassdoor, and Payscale.[18] Here is what they found:

1. The United States — $147,524
2. Australia – $134,000
3. Switzerland — $120,000
4. Israel — $84,000
5. Denmark — $93,000

6. Norway — $75,000
7. The United Kingdom — $75,000
8. Sweden — $73,000
9. The Netherlands — $80,000

The differences in CEO pay globally, according to Statista, were just as shocking.[19]

1. The United States — $14.25 million
2. Switzerland — $8.5 million
3. The Netherlands — $8.24 million
4. The United Kingdom — $7.95 million
5. Canada — $6.49 million
6. Germany — $6.27 million
7. Australia — $4.96 million
8. Spain — $4.89 million
9. Hong Kong — $4.88 million
10. Singapore — $4.62 million

Skilled workers in the U.S. make quite a bit more than in other countries. Period. Despite this, American physicians have been painted *en masse* as greedy and undeserving. If we are going to use such reasoning, then we must uniformly apply the same criteria across all professions, including American athletes.

IS THE SLICE OF PIE LARGE ENOUGH?

Regardless of where you stand on the doctor salary debate, the more important concern is whether it truly impacts the healthcare system in the long run. Economist Uwe Reinhardt has been arguing for the last decade that approximately 20% of American healthcare spending goes to physicians, with half of that earmarked for overhead including malpractice insurance.[20] Therefore, only about 10% of expenditures actually ends up in doctors' pockets.

Even if we were to halve their salaries, the impact on healthcare spending would be minimal. Coupled with the fact that physicians, along with dentists, shoulder the highest debt and have the highest suicide rates of any profession, the answer to whether doctors are being fairly compensated seems quite obvious: *No, they are not being paid enough.* This point is underscored by a 2022 AMA survey revealing that one in five physicians is planning to leave medicine in the next two years.[21]

WHAT HAPPENS WHEN TRUST IS LOST?

Due to the persistent narrative of painting doctors as responsible for our healthcare challenges, trust between doctors and patients is at an all-time low. According to a 2018 briefing by The Advisory Board citing a 2014 article in *The New England Journal of Medicine*, the proportion of Americans having confidence in their medical providers dropped from 75% in 1966 to as low as 34% today.[22] Moreover, Americans are less likely to trust their physicians compared to their peers in other developed nations.

This erosion of trust has transformed former allies into cautious adversaries and has real-time consequences. A *PloS One* article from 2017 examining these relationships came to the conclusion that, "*from a clinical perspective, patients reported more beneficial health behaviors, less symptoms and higher quality of life and to be more satisfied with treatment when they had higher trust in their health care professional.*" [23] Similarly, studies of patients who trust their doctors showed that they are more likely to take their medications, follow medical advice in general, and experience better mental and physical health. Conversely, those lacking trust are more likely to skip vaccinations.

A consequence of this distrust became glaringly obvious during the COVID pandemic. Widespread skepticism of the medical profession made adherence to basic health guidelines and obtaining preventative vaccinations far from guaranteed. This fallout led to a worsening of an already precarious situation. According to a 2021 survey by NORC at The University of Chicago commissioned by The American Board of Internal Medicine, as much as 30% of patients and doctors reported a decrease in their faith in our medical system due to the pandemic.[24]

We are grappling with an epidemic of mistrust.

This lack of trust generally originates from three primary drivers, as noted in Figure 1 from the NORC study.[24] The first is mostly about **competency.** Patients feel that doctors don't know them, listen to them, or fail to disclose all pertinent information. The resultant mistrust regarding

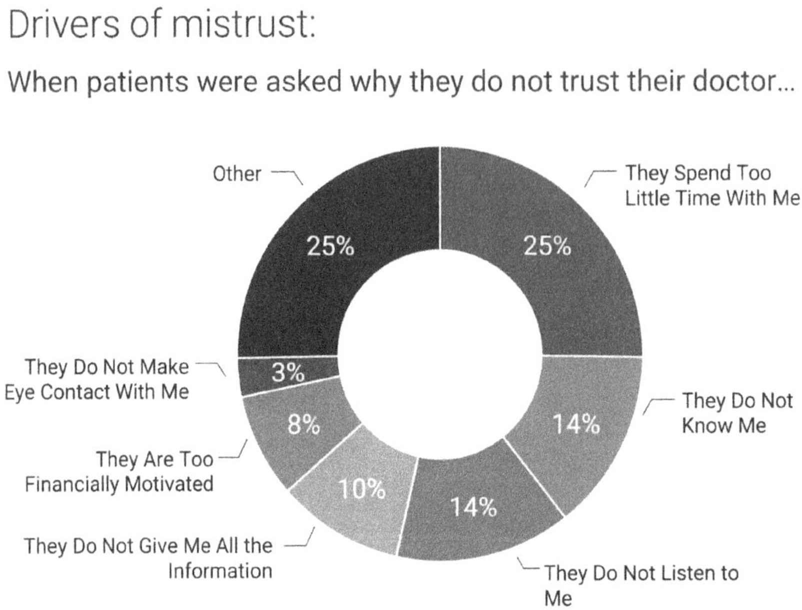

FIGURE 1. Drivers of Mistrust[24]

proficiency inevitably leads to engagement with the medicolegal system and malpractice.

The second driver involves **time.** Patients feel doctors spend too little time with them. A physicians' time is increasingly consumed by stringent compliance involved in record keeping, rather than being allocated to face-to-face care (access). This time has been exploited and weaponized by the powerful businesses that created electronic medical records.

The final driver is the belief that physicians are overly motivated by **financial considerations** (money). This perception is exacerbated by governmental reform that positions doctors as gatekeepers and by compliance pressures pushing our medical system into the embracing arms of venture capital, private equity, and big business.

In Part Two of this book, we will explore these topics further and delve into how external parties contribute to these faulty perceptions. But first, Chapter Two will take a look at some other non-provider-based ways in which patients have become nothing more than mere bargaining chips.

Before we move on, I want to highlight our humanity at the end of this chapter, as I will in every chapter.

Ultimately, as I will repeatedly emphasize, our society consists of those who need care and those who possess the necessary skills to deliver it. Everyone else is and should be superfluous. These vignettes tell their stories.

• • • • • •

I recall very few specific days from my first year of medical school amid the flood of facts, details, and minutia that mark the initial plunge into the depths of medical education. One memorable afternoon session stood out as part of our patient, physician, and society curriculum that was focused on embracing the biopsychosocial model of patient care — a precursor to what today is known as patient-centered care.

Sitting among my fellow students at the back of the classroom, we watched excitedly as the course director began the session with a viewing of the movie *The Doctor,* directed by Randa Haines and starring William Hurt.

Loosely based on Dr. Edward Rosenbaum's book *A Taste of My Own Medicine* (1988) the film's themes of compassion and empathy moved many of us to tears by the closing credits. It served as a powerful demonstration of how sensitivity toward patients can mold us into better doctors.

The Doctor/Dr. Edward Rosenbaum, Randa Haines, and William Hurt

In 1985, Dr. Edward Rosenbaum, a rheumatologist, received the diagnosis of throat cancer. During that tumultuous period, he kept a diary of his experiences which was later published by Penguin Random House under the title *A Taste of My Own Medicine*. This book served as the inspiration for the 1991 movie *The Doctor* and eventually become a best-seller.[25]

This collaborative storytelling effort between doctor, director, and actor helped remind audiences far and wide of how doctors and patients can collaborate in the process of disease management, and contributed to the acceptance of the biopsychosocial approach to care, initially described by George Engel in 1977.

In 2001 the Institute of Medicine spurred by their earlier report *To Err is Human* — a 1999 study documenting the profound effects of medical error — published *Crossing the Quality Chasm: A New Health System for the 21st Century*.[26] Among the new recommendations were six aims of healthcare quality. The third aim, dubbed patient-centered care, included the following description: "*Providing care that is respectful of and responsive to individual patient preferences, needs, and values and ensuring that patient values guide all clinical decisions*."

The retelling of Dr. Rosenbaum's story, as well as the Institute of Medicine's recommendations, have transformed the face of medical care. Medical schools across the country now include patient-centered care curriculums that focus on compassion, empathy, and the art of medical storytelling.

These bonds of allyship forged by patient-centered care were highlighted in a 2017 *NEJM Catalyst*[27] article for their role in achieving not only better individual care but also:

- Higher satisfaction scores among patients and their families.
- Enhanced reputation of providers among health care consumers.
- Improved morale and productivity among clinicians and ancillary staff.
- Optimized resource allocation.
- Reduced costs and increased financial viability across the care spectrum.

In sharing our stories, everyone benefits.

CHAPTER TWO.

Does a Spoonful of Sugar Really Help the Medicine Go Down?

SANTIAGO DIDN'T KNOW MUCH about medicine. He didn't understand why certain foods made his big toe swell and burn like it was sitting on a pile of hot coals. He had once been told that he had something called *gout*, which the doctor described as some sort of arthritis. But there was one thing that Santiago knew for sure: Taking a colchicine tablet daily, and three to four during attacks, saved him from an excruciating amount of pain.

Santiago couldn't afford insurance. While he made enough money to support his family with various short-term labor-intensive jobs, there wasn't much left over for luxuries. Fortunately, colchicine was available as a generic, costing him as little as $10 for a bottle of 30 tablets.

However, everything changed in September 2010 when the FDA mandated a halt on the manufacture, distribution, and marketing of unapproved single-ingredient oral colchicine under its Unapproved Drug Initiative.[1] Despite the fact that many of these formulations had been used safely in the United States for decades, they were removed because they had not undergone formal "modern-day FDA approval."

Unfortunately, only one company — URL Pharma — offered FDA-approved single-ingredient colchicine (Colcrys), and they promptly raised the price to $5 per pill. They justified the price increase by citing the cost of FDA approval, ongoing colchicine research (a drug used for decades), and the need for physician education.

Unable to afford to pay $150 for a month's supply, Santiago cut back and started taking a dose every other day to make the pills last. This change led to an increase in duration and severity of his gout flares, eventually resulting in hospitalization. The cost of hospital care and lost workdays quickly drained the little savings Santiago and his family had managed to accumulate. Even after all these hardships, he still faced the burden of the high monthly cost of this essential medication.

Adding injury to insult, URL Pharma was granted exclusive patent rights on Colcrys, a centuries-old medication, until 2029, limiting the number of generic alternatives whose price points were similar to the branded product.

A 2020 research letter published in the *Journal of the American Medical Association* reported that Medicaid spending on colchicine skyrocketed 2833% from 2008 to 2017.[1] In 2017, alone, Medicaid spending totaled $32 million, as compared to just $2.1 million if prices had not escalated due to the FDA approval issue.

Meanwhile, URL Pharma, whose sales of Colcrys soared to $430 million in 2011, was swiftly acquired by Takeda Pharmaceuticals for $800 million.[2] This acquisition delighted not only shareholders but also the Takeda C-suite, whose members were eagerly trying to diversify into America's expanding anti-inflammatory market. It seemed like a win for everybody — except, of course, Santiago, the broader American public, and doctors who lost access to an affordable medicine for a menacing and painful medical problem.

As Santiago's personal struggles demonstrate, the pharmaceutical industry has been fleecing the American public for decades. Their strategies include monopolizing product markets and creating new disease categories for which they offer seemingly perfect treatments. While their practices may be questionable, these companies frequently operate within legal boundaries and manage to avoid conflicts with regulatory bodies such as the FDA, which may be compromised by regulatory capture, which occurs when a regulatory agency that is supposed to act in the public interest becomes dominated or unduly influenced by the sector it is supposed to regulate.

Ultimately, these firms are channeling as much money as possible out of the American healthcare system and into their own pockets. Their justification hinges on the misguided belief that the only way to spur innovation is to promise a pot of gold at the end of what they consider to be an incredibly risky treasure hunt. They say that outsized profits are the cost of weighty research and development.

And they are mistaken!

THE RESEARCH AND DEVELOPMENT MYTH

Drug pricing in the United States is outrageously high. Yet, pharmaceutical companies repeatedly justify gouging patients like Santiago by citing the excessive cost of research and development. This was precisely the rationale URL Pharma used when raising the price of colchicine from mere pennies to just under $5 per pill.

On the surface, this argument seems logical. As noted by the Congressional Budget Office in 2021, the average cost to develop a new drug and bring it to market can range from $1 billion to $2 billion.[3] These costs are distributed evenly between discovery, development, testing, the cost of capitalization, and the expenses associated with approval and compliance.

Big Pharma has long maintained that reducing drug prices and the associated profits would severely hinder the development of new life-saving medications. Is that really the case?

Mo Money, Mo Problems?

Is Big Pharma truly generating more and better drugs by their heavily subsidized investment in research and development? Unfortunately, such simplistic explanations fail to capture the reality of how pharmaceutical companies are funded and how they allocate their precious resources.

As Richard Frank and Kathleen Hannick highlight in a 2022 article for the Brooking Institute, Big Pharma escalated its R&D spending from $37.5 billion in 2000 to $83 billion in 2019.[4] Despite this substantial increase, the rolling five-year average of new drug approvals rose only modestly, from 36.8 to 44 during the same period. They also noted that emerging biopharmaceutical firms, which spend less than $200 million annually for R&D, are responsible for over 80% of the pipeline projects from discovery to filing, compared to Big Pharma (global sales of $10 billion), which accounts for roughly 15%. The percentages have been steadily growing in favor of these smaller companies over the last decade.

Furthermore, the House Committee on Oversight and Reform has studied the biggest pharmaceutical companies and noted in 2019 that the 14 largest had R&D expenditures of $121 billion.[4] However, they observed that 10 out of 50 new drug applications that year came from only five of these companies; the other nine did not submit even one new drug application.

Nevertheless, you could still hypothesize that reducing pharmaceutical revenues by lowering drug costs could lead to the rapid decline in development of life-saving drugs. To address this question, Dranove and colleagues investigated the opposite scenario. They examined the impact of Medicare Part D, which expanded drug coverage and was a boon to Big Pharma's revenues, on the number of new drug launches. Their findings revealed that while there was an increase in the number of new drugs, most of them fell into the "me too" category.[5] These medications generally targeted therapeutic areas that already had at least five effective drugs, and thus very few were considered innovative. In other words, these "new" drugs cost Americans lots of money, but do little to improve on lesser-cost, already available, alternatives.

Finally, Frank and Hannick classified all FDA approvals from 2011 to 2021, categorizing them on whether they represented entirely new drugs, new combinations of existing drugs, or new indications for drugs already approved for other uses.[4] Shockingly, only 36% of these approvals involved totally new molecular formulations; the majority were essentially new packaging of old products.

Hey, Who Paid for That Anyway?

Another critical question arises when we consider public funding of pharmaceutical-backed research and development. In an *LA Times* op-ed entitled "How taxpayers prop up Big Pharma, and how to cap that," Mariana Mazzucato points out that "Since the 1930s, the National Institutes of Health has invested close to $900 billion in the basic and applied research that formed both the pharmaceutical and biotechnology sectors."[6]

Additionally, a report in the *Proceedings of the National Academy of Sciences* revealed that NIH funding contributed to published research associated with every single one of the 210 new drugs approved by the FDA from 2010 to 2016.[7] It's important to note, however, that the majority of this $900 billion is involved in basic science and bench research, which identifies drug targets rather than developing therapeutics.

While it is hard to deny that drug development and clinical trials are costly for Big Pharma, there is significant public funding for the foundational research on which these companies build their profitable products. The public, represented by everyday citizens, thus pays on the front end in terms of research and the back end through the high cost of pharmaceuticals.

Which raises an important question: What other perks and benefits does the pharmaceutical industry receive from the American public and the U.S. government?

Federal Perks, Credits, and Exclusivity

The government provides numerous tax credits and perks to encourage pharmaceutical companies to conduct research and develop new drugs. Foremost among these is a research and development tax credit, available to life sciences companies engaged in developing new drugs, biologics, devices, and more. This credit is accessible federally as well as in more than 30 states. Additionally, there is a separate orphan drug tax credit meant for companies developing treatments for rare diseases that affect smaller populations.

Furthermore, drug companies are fully allowed to deduct their costs for marketing and advertising, which amounted to an estimated $6 billion in deductions in 2015, as highlighted by Senator Claire McCaskill of Missouri, whose efforts to eliminate this deduction fell short in 2018.[8]

The most significant protection granted by the government to Big Pharma, however, is through laws that provide exclusivity through patenting. Patents typically last for 20 years from the filing date, but can be extended up to five more years based on the timing of clinical trials. Studies indicate that once a drug loses its patent protection, competition drives prices down by as much as 60%. Consequently, it is crucial for companies to ensure that their drugs never go off patent.

According to an investigation by I-MAK, the top 12 drugs on the market in 2018 were shielded by an unbelievable 848 patents, ensuring an average of 38 years without generic competition.[9] Many of the patent extensions were granted for new indications for treatment or minor modifications to the drug, such as combining it with another class of drugs to treat the same condition. I-MAK estimates that approximately 140 patents are filed for each major market-leading drug. And we have already seen how little of the profits created by these patents are actually being used to develop new drugs.

As noted in a 2017 *Harvard Business Review* article by Erin Fox, Big Pharma uses several tactics to protect their drugs.[10] For instance, according to the Federal Trade Commission, U.S. taxpayers and consumers bear an additional $3.5 billion in costs due to "pay-for-delay" tactics. This occurs when pharmaceutical companies pay generic manufacturers to postpone or even refrain from launching generic versions of their drugs.

Another strategy involves "citizen petitions" filed with the FDA that can delay generic drug production by as much as 150 days. Unsurprisingly, these petitions are often submitted by corporations rather than actual citizens, with drug manufacturers themselves responsible for as much as 92% of submissions.

While there is little doubt that the system is being manipulated, let's examine how these tactics unfold in real-time and adversely impact patients.

How Sweet It Is: Insulin and Oxycontin

The repercussions of pharmaceutical companies leveraging our healthcare system extends far beyond enriching their executives and shareholders; they are also having devastating consequences for the American people at large. Two drugs exemplify how the system is being gamed to benefit the few at the expense of the many.

Insulin

Prior to the Inflation Reduction Act in 2023, the rising cost of insulin had garnered prominent media attention since the beginning of the 21st century. Despite a 2022 study in *Health Affairs* showing that over 1.2 million Americans (14.1% of users) faced catastrophic spending levels on this all-important drug,[11] prices had surged by more than 300% over the last two decades.[12]

Remarkably, insulin, a drug in use for more than a century, has seen minimal innovation beyond alterations in duration and delivery systems — it generally works the same as it always has. This raises the important question of why drug prices haven't decreased. Why haven't advancements in manufacturing or generic competition placed downward pressure on the price for the average consumer?

The answers boil down to various strategies to extract wealth from the American people. A primary tactic, known as "evergreening," involves pharmaceutical companies modifying formulations to extend the patent of a profitable drug. This might entail slight modifications to alter bloodstream concentration or introduction of new drug delivery systems like injectable pen devices. These patent extensions and technological innovations hinder generic manufacturers from entering the market promptly. When patents do finally expire, the substantial cost associated with not only insulin manufacturing but also approval by U.S. regulators significantly deters most newcomers from entering the insulin market.[13]

Again, pharmaceutical companies often justify high prices by claiming they support further research, development, and innovation. However, they conveniently omit that the costs of modifying an existing medication or developing a new delivery method are significantly lower than those for creating, testing, and marketing a completely novel type of insulin.

Alarmingly, a new player has entered the fray in this brutal feeding frenzy. During a 2019 congressional hearing, insulin makers admitted to artificially maintaining high prices to appease pharmacy benefit managers.[12] These managers favor higher-priced medications because they yield greater overall profits. Companies like Eli Lilly run the risk of angering these intermediaries, potentially leading to exclusion from larger formularies and substantial loss of market share.

On a positive note, President Joe Biden's Inflation Reduction Act in 2023 imposed a cap on insulin costs at $35 per month for Medicare recipients.[14] Public outcry, along with Biden's strong advocacy in his State of the Union Address that year, prompted Eli Lilly to announce a 70% reduction in insulin prices and also the capping of out-of-pocket costs to the very same $35 per month.[15] Manufacturers Sanofi and Novo Nordisk quickly followed suit.

Oxycontin

The discussion of the pharmaceutical industry's detrimental impact on both the health and the pocketbooks of the American people would be incomplete without addressing oxycontin and the Sackler family. The three Sackler brothers, all physicians, owned Purdue Pharma and played key roles in formulating and aggressively marketing the highly addictive drug Oxycontin to patients and doctors.

The opioid epidemic has resulted in over 450,000 deaths over the last two decades.[15] Purdue Pharma was found guilty by the U.S. Department of Justice of conspiracy to defraud the United States and to violate the

Food, Drug, and Cosmetic Act, along with two counts of conspiracy to violate the federal anti-kickback statute.[16] Testimony revealed that Purdue misled the public about Oxycontin's addictive potential, utilized aggressive marketing techniques, and incentivized physicians to improperly prescribe this deadly drug.

Despite facing penalties and fines totaling over $6 billion — which bankrupted the parent company Purdue Pharma — the Sacklers themselves were shielded from personal liability. It is estimated that they diverted more than $10 billion into their accounts between 2004 and 2019.[17]

The end result was a $10 billion wealth transfer from the U.S. healthcare system into the hands of private individuals who not only lied, cheated, and stole, but also fueled a public health crisis that will incur billions more for acute and chronic care of addicted individuals, as well as create the need for new and costly public health initiatives.

Disease Mongering

The pharmaceutical industry not only capitalizes on the current state of medical care to raise drug prices and maintain its monopoly but also engages in a far more covert strategy to strip the public of much-needed healthcare resources. The term disease mongering[18] was first coined to describe the process by which Big Pharma uses marketing and advertising to invent new diseases and subsequently offers expensive medications to treat them.[19] Disease mongering employs various tactics in order to maximize profits:

- Medicalizing ordinary or non-pathological conditions, such as medications for obesity and baldness.
- Aggressively treating pre-disease states, such as the preventative use of statin medications for cholesterol or oral diabetes medications for "pre-diabetes."
- Treating risk factors as diseases themselves, such as promoting daily use of aspirin to prevent coronary disease or calcium supplements to prevent osteoporosis.

Pharmaceutical companies aggressively promote these states as pathological through direct-to-consumer advertising, sales presentations masked as "continuing education" in physicians' offices, and through the creation of socially savvy disease awareness campaigns, all aimed at boosting product sales. They often exaggerate effectiveness, encourage off-label use by physicians, and lower diagnostic thresholds, all in pursuit of increasing profits.[20]

Many, in fact, would argue that disease mongering was instrumental in the rise of Oxycontin and Purdue Pharma. By medicalizing everyday occurrences such as physical pain, they turned these "symptoms" into opportunities to increase narcotic sales. What was once considered the common aches and pains of life became marketed as new diseases states that could be treated with expensive and ultimately deadly pharmaceuticals.

Pharmaceutical sales representatives fanned out across the nation, visiting doctors in their own offices and emphasizing the urgency of treating a new mysterious "epidemic of pain." The solution, they said, was as simple as prescribing a few "non-addicting" Oxycontin pills. Physician influencers and key opinion leaders who can sway public opinion were enticed into *educating* their peers on easing opioid prescription guidelines by offering them substantial consulting fees. Purdue Pharma became a major source of physician training programs and even launched international pain awareness campaigns.[21]

While the Sackler family amassed billions, the health of Americans deteriorated, hundreds of thousands died, and the costs to address this terrifying opioid crisis, a crisis they helped create, skyrocketed. Pharmaceutical companies are laughing their way to the bank while the rest of us suffer. And have no doubt, those corporate bank accounts are growing at an exponential rate.

THE RISING PROFITABILITY OF PHARMACEUTICAL COMPANIES

The pharmaceutical industry in the United States is thriving. According to testimony at a hearing before the U.S. Senate's Committee on Finance in May 2023, the top seven pharmaceutical giants (AbbVie, Amgen, Bristol Myers Squibb, Eli Lilly, Gilead, Johnson & Johnson, Merck, and Pfizer) amassed $110 billion in profits in 2022, marking a breathtaking 104% increase from the year prior.[22] Astonishingly, according to this same hearing, these companies paid a paltry $2 billion in total taxes on these enormous profits.

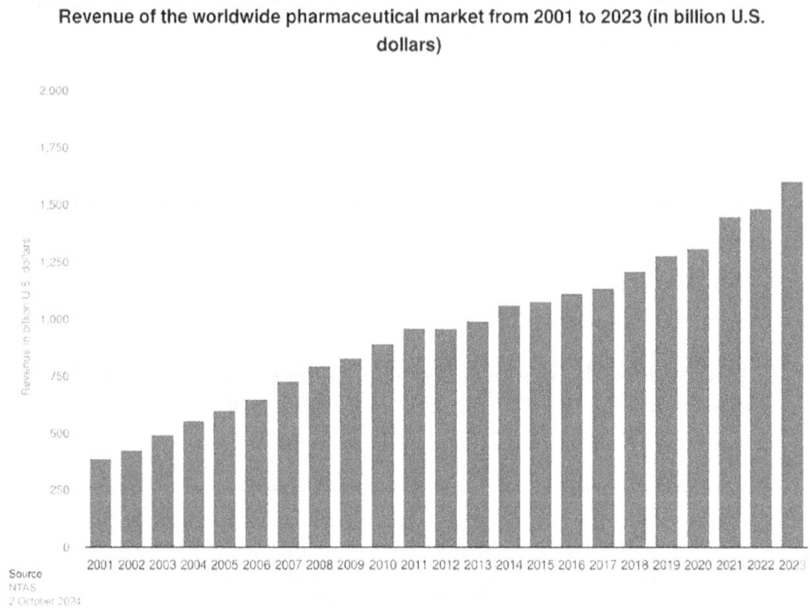

FIGURE 2. Revenue of the worldwide pharmaceutical market from 2001 to 2023 (in billion U.S. dollars). (Statista 2023).

AbbVie, who stands out as one of the most egregious, reported losses of $5 billion domestically and $20 billion internationally in 2022. Despite the fact that most of its profits come from the domestic sale of its arthritis drug Humira, the company has reported losses every year in the United States since 2013.[23] How does AbbVie manage to stay afloat? Somehow the company still was able to pay its CEO Richard Gonzalez a hefty $25.7 million in 2023.[23] In fact, CEOs of 13 of the top pharmaceutical companies collectively earned over $1 billion in total compensation.[24]

As mentioned previously, according to the Governmental Accountability Office,[25] among the 25 largest pharmaceutical companies, the average profit margin fluctuated between 15% and 20%. This starkly contrasts with the annual average profit margin of non-drug companies in the S&P 500, which typically ranges between 4% and 9%. Globally, as illustrated in Figure 2, pharmaceutical revenue in 2023 was estimated at $1.6 trillion, a significant leap from $390 billion in 2001. Over a quadrupling in 22 years.[26]

The Price Fix Is In!

Santiago, our patient with gout, is not alone in facing tough decisions when it comes to medicine and affordability. Research indicates that prescription prices in the United States are often as much as two to four times those in other industrialized countries.[27] Another report analyzing 2019 data found that spending on prescription medications in the United States was $1,126 per person, surpassing spending in all other comparable countries.[28]

The reasons behind these outrageous expenditures are glaringly evident. As with colchicine and insulin, pharmaceutical companies justify price gouging by citing the costs of research and development, a cost that is heavily subsidized by the public. Additionally, they benefit from federal perks and extended patents. Adding insult to injury, these companies create new disease processes through disease mongering while deceiving the American public and the U.S. government about the effectiveness and safety of their products. These deceptive practices not only cost us trillions of dollars but have also contributed to public health crises such as the opioid epidemic sparked by drugs like Oxycontin.

Despite doctors often being blamed for rising healthcare costs due to overtreatment or selecting costly drugs and equipment, a recent survey showed that 73% of doctors indicated they consider patients' out-of-pocket costs while making clinical decisions.[29] As medication prices escalate, many still attribute rising costs to "Cowboy Doctors" who are just "out to make a buck."[30]

The price fix is in and doctors and patients alike have merely become the instrument of corporate profits. Sadly, as we will see in the next few chapters, pharmaceutical companies are not the only ones who are using these shameful tactics.

TOWARD BUILDING A BETTER SYSTEM

While the challenges facing the pharmaceutical industry are widespread, they are not completely insurmountable. Several commonsense solutions could be implemented through effective legislation to balance the incentives of pharmaceutical industry profitability with the necessity of more reasonable and fair drug prices. Though not exhaustive, the following recommendations could have an immediate impact.

Patent Reform

One of the most obvious hurdles to reducing drug prices is the extended exclusivity of production granted through patent laws. In the United States, current patent regulations allow pharmaceutical companies lengthy periods to monopolize production, distribution, and pricing of new drugs. Patent protection should be revised to shorten these periods and restrict companies from repeatedly extending them for minor modifications or new indications within already crowded drug classes. This would restrict patent protection to cover only truly innovative medications that offer a substantially new clinical benefit.

Faster Generic Approval

The generic approval process in the United States is frequently slow and often discouraging. When a generic manufacturer identifies a drug nearing patent expiration, there is typically a 30-month delay for litigation to determine if the patent has truly expired. This stay lasts until all litigation is concluded.[31] Moreover, even after all that, the first generic manufacturer has a 180-day period of exclusivity before other companies can begin producing the same medication.[32] These procedural bottlenecks cost the American people billions of dollars and are readily amenable to legislative reform.

Value-Based Price Capping

Almost every new cancer drug introduced in the United States in the past few years has surpassed the $100,000 mark, with the median price reaching as high as $150,000 in 2018.[33] Despite the fact that many of these drugs are either appropriate for a small subset of patients or offer marginal improvements over the benefits of pre-existing therapies, there is no legislated cap on the cost of new drugs in America. This lack of regulation particularly effects the drugs' value relative to their impact on the population. Implementing value-based caps could significantly reduce the prices of some of the most expensive drugs.

Medicare Negotiation

Simply put, Medicare is one the biggest purchasers of prescription drugs in the United States. However, the Medicare Prescription Drug,

Improvement, and Modernization Act of 2003 expressly prohibits the Secretary of Health and Human Services from negotiating Medicare prices or establishing a preferred drug formulary.[34] One study showed that if Medicare negotiated drug prices for VA care only, there would be a savings of more than $14.4 billion.[35]

In 2022, Congress passed the Inflation Reduction Act (IRA) which, for the first time, authorizes the Secretary of the Department of Health and Human Services (HHS) to negotiate prices directly with participating manufacturers for some high expenditure, qualifying, single-source drugs without generic competition.[35] While this represents a positive step forward, billions of dollars are still being left on the table.

Price Inflation

The United States lacks price caps on brand name drugs, which often results in unchecked cost inflation. As illustrated with insulin and colchicine, prices of previously affordable drugs can skyrocket seemingly without justification. Between 2012 and 2017, the United States spent $6.8 billion in excess solely due to price increases in pre-existing brand name cancer medications, while the rest of the world collectively saved $1.7 billion on the same drugs over the same period.[36]

While these recommendations will not entirely resolve the pharmaceutical industries cost issues, they will go a long way toward curbing the currently unchecked system. Despite anticipated resistance from these highly profitable companies, leveraging the current bevy of federal perks and incentives could certainly ensure compliance with these much-needed reforms.

• • • • • •

Any doctor who practiced in an office-based setting at the turn of this century can vividly recall countless interactions with pharmaceutical representatives. They would arrive at our practice several days a week bearing lunch for the whole staff, glossy brochures for each of the physicians, and a wealth of research extolling the virtues of whichever drug they were promoting that day.

Over the years, while the names of the drugs changed frequently, the tactics remained consistent. Despite many of us being skeptical of the selectively presented material, the free drug samples they left behind to dispense to our cash-strapped patients undeniably influenced our prescription choices.

Often there were also thinly veiled offers to work for the company as part of a speaker's bureau. There were attempts to incentivize us to not only increase the number of prescriptions we wrote but also to become key thought leaders among our peers and colleagues. While many of us remained vigilant of these attempts to sway our behavior, numerous studies have documented an uptick in prescription rates following visits from drug representatives.[37]

One physician decided to shine a light on these unethical practices.

Overdosed America: The Broken Promise of American Medicine/John Abramson

John Abramson, after 20 years of caring for his small-town community north of Boston, found that his role as a caregiver was being undermined by increasing pressure to prescribe the latest drugs and adopt the most up-to-date but expensive technology for almost every problem. His disillusionment led to the confrontation between two warring factions: the desire to improve his patient's health versus the goal of optimizing profits. In his book *Overdosed America*, Abramson meticulously exposes how commercial interests distort the information upon which doctors and patients alike rely.[38]

Through powerful storytelling and patient anecdotes, Abramson writes about how his journey began with the profound and disappointing realization that the benefits of a whole family of medicines, the Cox-2 inhibitors (Celebrex and Vioxx among others), had largely been exaggerated through aggressive marketing materials and industry-backed studies aimed at boosting sales.

Moreover, Abramson argues that such aggressive marketing not only drives unnecessary demand but also drives a wedge between doctors and patients while eroding trust. This loss of trust is not only limited to the economic fallout but also can have a deleterious effect on patient outcomes. The author, at one point, mourns how aggressive marketing pushed the overutilization of a class of medications called "anti-arrhythmics," which, despite initial promises, ended up causing more harm than good. How many lives were unnecessarily lost?

One of the most enduring lessons from Abramson's work is the reminder that basic health behaviors — such as an appropriate diet, exercise, and avoiding smoking — are still the cornerstones of well-being. He emphasized that these lifestyle changes are often cheaper, more effective, and less harmful than the costly drugs that have been so heavily thrust upon us by Big Pharma.

CHAPTER THREE.

How Sure Are You About Insurance?

MARYBETH HAD PAID REMARKABLY LITTLE ATTENTION to her health insurance until now. The policy provided through the medical practice that she managed had been fairly generous thus far. She regularly paid the modest monthly premiums, and all acute and yearly preventative care for her husband and her was covered.

When her husband Jim showed up one morning in her office unable to smile or move one side of his face, Marybeth found solace in knowing that he would receive care from the very best doctors at the hospital across the street from her practice, with all expenses covered by their insurance policy. This small oasis of hope sustained her during Jim's tumultuous two weeks in the hospital where magnetic resonance imaging of the brain revealed that he had suffered an acute stroke. Given Jim's young age — he was only 40 at the time — a search for underlying causes was undertaken.

The cardiologist, a familiar face to Marybeth from her years as an office manager in an internal medicine practice, expressed optimism when he explained the findings of Jim's cardiac echocardiogram. The hole in Jim's heart, a condition known as a patent foramen ovale (or PFO) was likely the culprit causing his premature stroke, and a medical procedure seemed to be a straightforward solution to his condition.

Marybeth consulted all the doctors in her office and found unanimous agreement with the treatment plan, but was warned that the research regarding his situation was still evolving. While the procedures and devices for closing a PFO had been available since the early 2000s, the evidence supporting their effectiveness was still emerging. Despite this, however, her colleagues felt a great deal of confidence in the cardiologist's recommendation, believing that the procedure needed to be performed.

Now this wasn't Marybeth's first rodeo. She had spent hours on the phone with insurance companies as a medical office manager and knew that reimbursement for procedures could be precarious. Following her own advice to the practice's patients, she contacted her insurer, explained the situation to the customer service operator, and requested a coverage determination. To her great surprise, the operator assured her that the procedure had already been preapproved.

With great relief, Jim underwent the procedure, recovered smoothly, and after a brief stay in a rehabilitation facility, returned back to his previous life, functioning normally. Marybeth was grateful not only for the excellent medical care Jim received but also for the insurance coverage that supported it. Little did she know that a few months later, a new nightmare would begin.

Upon receiving a letter from her insurer, Marybeth was perplexed by the legal jargon but not the overall intent of the correspondence. Despite the prior authorization of Jim's procedure, the insurer now was issuing a retroactive denial, deeming the closure of a patent foramen ovale too experimental for coverage. Consequently, they decided not to reimburse the hospital or doctors, leaving Marybeth and her husband with a daunting $50,000 bill to pay out of pocket. When Marybeth pointed out the prior authorization, the insurance company kindly directed her to a singular clause buried within dense legal language that stated that "prior authorization is not a guarantee of future payment."

Marybeth was devastated. How could she, in the midst of one of the biggest crises of her life, go against the advice of her trusted doctors and decline a surgery that she could have only learned might not be covered if she had meticulously read and understood all the details in a random statement sent to her home? The deck was stacked against her. It is stacked against us all.

Years later, after finally settling the last of the $50,000 debt owed to the medical center, Marybeth remains steadfast in her belief that the care Jim received was not only appropriate but also likely life-saving. She would give anything to make sure that Jim never had a stroke again. Her faith in insurance companies, however, was irreparably damaged.

As of the writing of this book, additional research has emerged and multiple recommendations support PFO closure in situations similar to Jim's to now be the standard of care.[1] Jim's doctors likely provided lifesaving treatment, affirming Marybeth's decision to pursue the procedure for her husband's well-being. Jim remains healthy today.

Conversely, the insurer was mistaken in denying care coverage and ultimately saved $50,000. It's worth noting that this insurer has achieved record-breaking profits every year since then.

HEALTH INSURANCE: A MASSIVE WEALTH TRANSFER

Marybeth and Jim's experience is not unique. The health insurance industry has adopted techniques to hinder access to care upfront, deny payment after the fact, and continuously hike premiums exponentially. Their tactics range from imposing cumbersome preapproval processes for medicines and procedures, to arbitrary and often retroactive claims denial. Doctors find themselves inundated in paperwork, navigating labyrinth-like phone trees, and often forced into the backbreaking work of fighting for patients' rights after denials. Drug formularies, crucial for prescribing medications, are difficult to locate, frequently updated, and manipulated to optimize insurers' profits while causing maximum inconvenience to doctors and patients alike.

Despite legislative efforts like the Affordable Care Act, which aimed to expand healthcare access, unintended consequences have emerged. As highlighted in Chapter One, federal regulations now cap insurers' profits as a percentage of total expenditures on care. This means insurers earn more as they spend more, removing the incentive to negotiate cost-effective care. Each time the cost of a procedure or medication rises, insurers willingly pay more knowing it boosts their bottom line — funded by higher premiums charged to customers.

Instead of safeguarding the health and safety of Americans, the insurance business has become a massive wealth transfer from citizens' pockets and into the bank accounts of these large corporations. For many, like Marybeth and Jim, who have faithfully paid insurance premiums for decades, accessing high-quality care often means bearing the financial burden all by themselves.

In Denial Over Denials

It is one of the single most important questions consumers ask when they are deciding on health insurance policies: *"Will this policy cover what my doctors say is necessary?"*

This question weighed heavily on Marybeth's mind as she deliberated with her practice's doctors and picked a health insurance policy a few months before Jim unexpectedly had a stroke. Yet, for the average consumer, obtaining this type of information is all but impossible. As noted by *ProPublica* in 2023, only two states collect and publicize such data, but it's limited to a small subset of health plans covering a minimal number of people.[2]

Despite the Affordable Care Act in 2010 granting federal regulators greater authority to compel insurers to disclose denial data, more than a decade later, much of this critical information is still not forthcoming. While there have been instances of insurers specifically targeting individuals' costly claims for heightened scrutiny,[3] the inner workings of the coverage process largely remain opaque to the public.

The Kaiser Family Foundation originally sought to shed light on the nature of these denials by analyzing transparency data provided by the Centers for Medicare & Medicaid Services through a public use file. Their analysis revealed that in 2020, out of the 230.9 million in-network claims received for patients covered under the Healthcare Marketplace at healthcare.gov, 42.3 million were denied — an average in-network claims denial rate of 18.3%.[4] That means almost one in five claims was rejected!

Upon reevaluation of the same data in 2024, Kaiser found a similar overall denial rate of 20%.[5] Because CMS requires insurers to categorize and explain the reasons for their decisions, we are able to glean deeper insights from the data: 5% were denied due to a lack of medical necessity as determined by the insurer (akin to Marybeth and Jim's experience), 36% for reason not listed, 25% were based on administrative reasons, and 9% for a lack of prior authorization or referral.

Further examining Medicare Advantage programs in 2021, Kaiser discovered that over 2 million prior-authorization forms were either partially or fully denied, with only 11% of these denials being appealed; 82% of those appealed were either partially or fully overturned,[6] underscoring the challenges and disparities in the initial claim processing within these programs.

Claims appeals and denial data for healthcare.gov consumers for 2021 paints an equally grim picture. Kaiser's analysis revealed that individuals appealed fewer than two-tenths of 1% of denied in-network claims, with only about a 40% chance of success.[7]

As Jessica Roy highlighted in the *LA Times* in 2022,[8] "Fighting an insurance company can be exhausting. Health insurers often make appeals and reimbursement processes difficult.... For many people, it may be less taxing to give up and accept a different treatment or medication, pay out of pocket, or go without treatment altogether, than to expend the energy fighting with their health plan."

Private insurers are using preauthorization, inappropriate denials, and delay tactics, capitalizing on the assumption that many consumers will either passively accept their decisions or eventually lose this battle of attrition.

The Problem with Preauthorization

Consumer frustrations with prior or preauthorizations are widespread in the U.S. healthcare system. Research shows that 16% of all insured adults experienced a prior authorization issue within the last year.[7] The burden was even more pronounced among individuals with conditions such as mental illness, diabetes, and those requiring more frequent healthcare services — in other words, the very groups most at risk for costly and poor healthcare outcomes.

Furthermore, the same survey revealed significant consequences of these authorization problems. Patients facing insurance hurdles, including prior authorizations, were three times more likely to report being unable to access medical care or treatment recommended by their healthcare provider. They were also twice as likely to report a decline in their health due to these barriers, with a third reporting increased out-of-pocket expenses.

While it is understandable that insurance companies are using prior authorizations to try to control costs, as reported by the American Medical Association,[9] the outcomes for patients can be devastating.

- **It complicates decision making**: Choosing the right procedures and medications tailored to a patient's unique medical needs is already complex. Each decision requires several considerations, including cost, side-effect profile, and interactions with other treatments and medications. Adding to this problem is the prior-authorization process, where doctors often lack the most up-to-date information on which medications will require prior approval in the first place. Sometimes, patients don't find out about these requirements until they reach the pharmacy.

- **The rules are unclear**: "For the medications or procedures that do require prior authorization, it's a bit of a guessing game. We don't actually know what piece of information the health insurer is looking for, so we send a bunch of explanations," according to Dr. Jack Resneck. "But if it doesn't exactly match what the health plan employee is looking for on their computer screen, then oftentimes it won't get approved — even if it's justified and evidence-based."[9]
- **Fighting rejections is time consuming**: Practices complete, on average, 39 authorizations per physician per week.[10] Physicians and their staff members spend an average of 13 hours weekly on these requests. Approximately 40% of physicians have staff who work exclusively on prior authorizations; 89% of physicians said that prior authorizations somewhat or significantly increase physician burnout.
- **Real harm is happening**: Adverse outcomes are more common when medications are delayed or not filled at all; many patients caught in the prior authorization maze never receive their medications. The process also strains the doctor-patient relationship, eroding trust when physicians and staff are unable to navigate the process or are unaware of the barriers patients will face once they leave the office.
- **An everchanging landscape**: The prior-authorization process is in constant flux. Insurers frequently update formularies at irregular intervals, subjecting long-term medication users to new authorization requirements. The unpredictability delays care and frustrates both doctors and patients.

Encouragingly, both federal and state governments have continued to take action on prior authorization reform. As of 2024, nine states had enacted legislation addressing prior authorization, with more than 90 bills introduced across 30 states. Since then, momentum has accelerated — at least 10 states passed additional reforms during the 2024 legislative session, and by 2025, at least 18 states had taken new legislative or regulatory action.[11] Furthermore, CMS finalized a rule in January 2024 to modernize and streamline the prior-authorization process for various programs, including Medicare Advantage.[11] Some states are also challenging retroactive denials,[12] such as the one Jim and Marybeth encountered.

You Pay a Premium

Possibly one of the most frustrating aspects of the ongoing denials of care and the prior authorization process is that consumers continue paying premiums to companies that try to hinder them every time they try to use their benefits. And those premiums, an utter surprise to no one, continue to rise steadily.

According to a 2023 employer health benefits survey, average annual premiums reached $8,435 for single coverage and $23,968 for family coverage, marking an increase of 7% from the previous year.[13] Average family premiums have surged by 22% since 2018 and 47% since 2013. These premiums are projected to rise to unprecedented levels in the future.[14]

The various factors that lead to these rising costs include medical inflation, an aging population, technological advances, and increased administrative overhead and governmental compliance. More striking, however, is that health insurers as an industry are unwilling to use their size and purchasing power to drive down costs.

As highlighted by Robert Pearl in his 2023 *Forbes* article,[15] more than half of Americans (169 million) are covered by the big five insurers: UnitedHealth Group, Anthem (now Elevance), Aetna, Cigna, and Humana. Private insurance is a $1.2 trillion-a-year industry that accounts for 30% of all healthcare spending. In a healthcare landscape dominated by monopolies in pharmaceuticals and hospital systems, the insurance sector is arguably the largest.

Given the power and size of these five companies, one would expect them to leverage their influence to negotiate better prices for their customers and reduce healthcare costs. However, insurance companies have taken a rather laissez-faire approach. Instead of actively striving to optimize care and reduce costs, as Pearl noted in his *Forbes* article,[15] they tend to adopt a more actuarial approach. This means they calculate the expected costs — regardless of how inflated they may be — and then adjust the premiums accordingly, rather than actively seeking systemic improvements.

Indeed, under the Affordable Care Act, insurers are required to issue rebates and lower premiums if they spend less than 80% of collected premiums on medical care. There is no incentive, however, for them to do this. When insurers pay less for services, medications, or procedures, their profits decrease accordingly.

This setup creates a win-win scenario for everyone except the patients who are stuck footing the bill. Pharmaceutical and device companies inflate their prices, hospital systems raise their rates for procedures and hospital stays, and insurance companies collect higher premiums and pay out even more for medical care. And everyone is laughing all the way to the bank. Meanwhile patients, of course, bear the financial burden necessary to fund all these third parties.

A similar pattern emerges with medical fraud. As a result of insurers' extensive data and the large number of lives covered, it would seem appropriate for them actively to root out fraudulent medical providers in order to create a better, more efficient healthcare system. Yet as Marshall Allen writes in *ProPublica* in 2019, sparingly little fraud is pursued or litigated by the big five health insurers.[16] In many cases, they avoid these investigations due to the low short-term return on investment, and the necessity of maintaining large and well-organized physician networks available for their customers to access.

Instead of cracking down on fraud, insurance companies pass on costs and lost revenue to their customers. We all pay the bill. Meanwhile insurers continue to enjoy soaring profits.

Together, these factors contribute to the ongoing increase in premiums.

It Pays to Insure

Up to this point, we have discussed how the system has been intentionally structured to maximize profits for the health insurance industry while using minimal resources, and leaving the public to foot the bill. The real question, however, is: How successful have they been? The answer, unfortunately, is quite shocking.

Over the past decade, health insurance companies have experienced explosive growth. The top six for-profit companies alone now account for over 30% of all healthcare spending,[17] significantly up from a just 10% as recently as 2011. Yet this growth in total revenues doesn't tell the whole

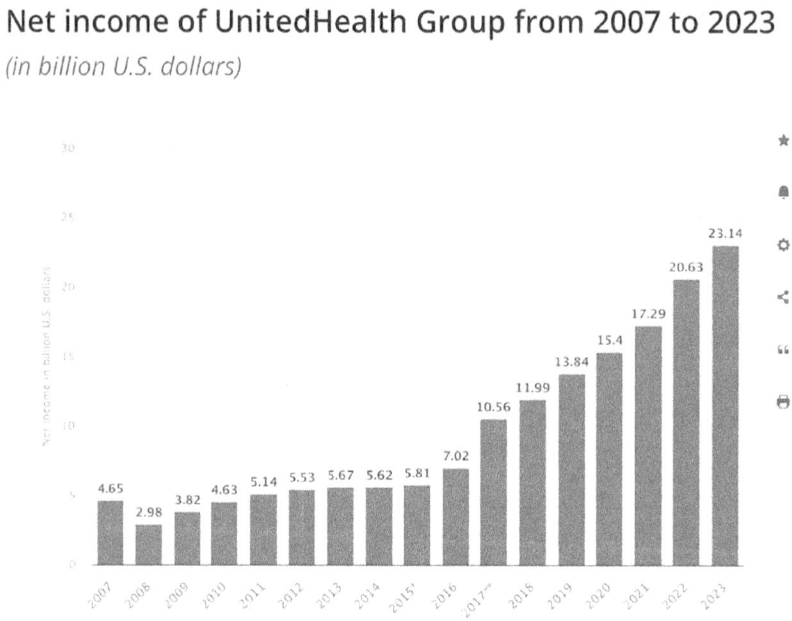

FIGURE 3. Net Income of UnitedHealth Group.[18]

story. One could argue that the insurers, like the American public, are victims of rampant cost inflation and are merely raising premiums in order to cover increasingly expensive expenditures. Maybe, despite some of the underhanded tactics we have already described in this chapter, these massive conglomerates are facing challenges similar to those affecting everyone else.

To explore this question further, let's delve deeper into the poster child for the health insurance industry: United Healthcare.

As is evident in Figure 3, net income has surged nearly 500% over the past decade.[18] This record profitability has enabled the company to allocate a staggering $23.5 million in total compensation to CEO Andrew Witty for 2023 alone. While United Healthcare leads in profits, CVS Health ($8.3 billion), Elevance Health ($6 billion), and Cigna Group ($5.2 billion) are also thriving on their own and continue to experience rapid growth.

When it comes to the health insurance industry, the recipe for success is clear: higher premiums and lower payouts. The well-being of the public remains missing from the calculation.

TOWARD BUILDING A BETTER SYSTEM

There are undoubtedly numerous solutions, both immediate and incremental, to address the challenges of our for-profit health insurance system. While some proposals, such as universal coverage funded by the government and our taxes, are considered extreme, there are also some less aggressive changes that could yield positive outcomes without dismantling our current free-market approach.

Universal Basic Coverage

One of the most radical solutions proposed is universal basic healthcare coverage, in which insurance is removed from the business realm and becomes a government-funded benefit of citizenship. As Amy Finkelstein and Liran Einav argue, the most viable way of moving forward may be universal basic healthcare coverage that provides access to essential healthcare regardless of the insured's resources.[19] They contend that since taxpayers already foot the bill when individuals' healthcare costs go unpaid — with half of total costs already being taxpayer financed, amounting to about 9% of GDP — citizens are spending as much as most other countries' governments do on universal health.

Align Incentives

As discussed earlier in this chapter, there is a critical need for better alignment between health insurers and the good of the American public regarding the delivery of low-cost care. Currently, these large companies have multiple reasons to overspend on drugs, equipment, procedures, and hospital stays, passing on these inflated costs to consumers in the form of increased premiums. This not only boosts insurers' profits but also diminishes their incentive to combat fraud or negotiate aggressively with pharmacy benefit managers to lower costs.

Price Transparency

With the proliferation of high deductibles, copays, and health savings accounts, consumers now have stronger incentives than ever to price-compare for "shoppable" medical supplies and services. For example, choosing one medical center over another for a hip replacement can significantly affect out-of-pocket costs. A 2025 federal fact sheet cited analyses suggesting that price transparency initiatives proposed by the Trump administration could generate savings of up to $80 billion in 2025 alone. [20]

However, a major obstacle remains: The average consumer often lacks access to clear information about what medical procedures will cost. Not only are the prices for common procedures hard to find, but charges can vary widely on a fee-for-service basis, depending on the resources utilized during a given hospitalization or procedure.

Although federal law has mandated hospitals to publicly disclose pricing and discount rates for common health services since 2021, an analysis by the Kaiser Family Foundation in 2023 found the data to be "messy, inconsistent and confusing, making it challenging, if not impossible, for patients or researchers to use them for their intended purpose."[21]

If we want to improve this situation, we must prioritize the public's access to critical pricing information. We can't do better unless we know more.

......

As a busy practicing physician, I found few tasks more exasperating than dealing with insurance companies. I often spent countless hours filling out prior authorizations, responding to repetitive phone queries, and witnessing my patients' struggle with the financial burden of their premiums, copays, and deductibles. Requests from insurance companies were often illogical, redundant, and exhausting.

Treatments that had been proven to work for patients for years suddenly became nonformulary or were moved into a higher copay tier. Essential medical tests and procedures were often denied, despite strong endorsements of medical necessity by both primary care doctors and specialists. And infuriatingly, sudden changes in provider networks left patients paying out of network fees for physicians they had known and worked with for a lifetime.

Meanwhile, low-paid insurance company employees often blamed physicians for these and other issues:

- *"If your doctor hadn't left our network. . . ."*
- *"If your doctor had filled out the prior authorization correctly. . . ."*
- *"If your doctor would just stop ordering these unnecessary tests. . . ."*

As a physician, it became abundantly clear to me that the insurance companies were engaged in a concerted propaganda war not only against doctors, but also against reform-minded politicians and anyone else who posed a threat to their increasing profits.

There is one person, however, who was willing to bravely stand in their path. Previously considered to be one of their very own, Wendall Potter, once part of the insurance industry, chose to blow the whistle on his former colleagues.

And he did so through storytelling.

Deadly Spin: An Insurance Company Insider Speaks Out on How Corporate PR Is Killing Healthcare and Deceiving Americans/Wendall Potter.

In June 2009, Wendall Potter delivered groundbreaking testimony before the Senate panel on healthcare reform, delivering a stunning blow to the health insurance industry. A former vice president at Cigna, he exposed how health insurers manipulate the system with little regard for patients, regulations, or the general well-being of our healthcare system.

In his book *Deadly Spin*, Potter takes us behind the scenes, revealing how funds diverted from healthcare are used for political lobbying as well as a propaganda campaign aimed at undermining any threat to their immense profits.[22] These tactics include fabricating scientific studies, creating bogus grassroot organizations, and even inventing catchy slogans (such as *Death Panels*) adopted by sympathetic politicians to defeat consumer-focused legislation.

While Potter's congressional appearance and book did not revolutionize the system and lead to immediate and drastic change, they did catalyze major reforms that were included in the Affordable Care Act in 2010. Today, he leads The Center for Health and Democracy (CHD) which is a nonprofit organization dedicated to reforming America's system of health coverage.

CHAPTER FOUR.

Is Healthcare Any of Your Business?

THE RISE OF ELECTRONIC MEDICAL RECORDS, Medicare audits, and a growing emphasis on compliance have prompted private practitioners, medical groups, and hospital systems alike to look for swift and lucrative escape hatches. According to *Kaiser Health News*, private equity had one of its best years in 2021, pouring more than $206 billion into 1,400 healthcare acquisitions, spanning the gamut that includes eye clinics, dental chains, and physician practices, among others.[1] Private equity is a type of investment that involves buying and managing companies that are not publicly traded or listed on a stock exchange.

KHN's investigation, however, also reveals a darker side of such acquisitions: Companies owned or managed by private equity have incurred over $500 million in fines since 2014 and have been forced to settle at least 34 lawsuits filed under the False Claims Act — a federal law that targets false billing submissions to the federal government and calls for substantial fines.[2]

Notably, we face an ethical cliff as ownership transfers from physicians and other healthcare providers to private corporate entities. While lacking enforcement, many practitioners recite, internalize, and practice by moral standards of conduct such as the Hippocratic Oath or the Oath of Geneva. These oaths forge a profound bond between doctor and patient — one that transcends mere business obligations such as due diligence to shareholders. Doctors are not obligated to prioritize financial gain for anyone. Corporate entities, on the other hand, swear to and operate by no such oaths.

STANDARDS OF CARE

The corporatization of healthcare is evident to anyone working in the trenches, striving to deliver exceptional care to those in need. When I began my career as a hospice physician in 2010, I joined a physician-owned hospice that not only upheld the highest standards of care but also prioritized patient and family comfort. Our chief medical officer, an engaged practicing physician, consistently shared case studies and the most up-to-date research, fostering a culture of continuous medical education within our practice of physicians and nurses.

Subsequently, our hospice merged with two others to create a much larger corporate entity. In an effort to manage escalating administrative costs, popular patient services such as massage and music therapy were diminished and eventually completely cut. Years later, a Medicare audit revealed compliance lapses in the original merger, resulting in hefty fines of several million dollars that severely impacted our hospice's financial health. Despite being one of the area's largest hospices, the fines dealt an incredible blow to the bottom line, leading to what could only be considered a fire sale to a major private equity firm with numerous healthcare interests.

The transfer of ownership brought stark changes for me as a physician. Years earlier, our medical team had conducted a review on the usage of medications to control secretions in end-of-life care. End-of-life secretions, also known as terminal respiratory secretions or "death rattle," are a natural part of the dying process for many people who are terminally ill. Based on our findings, which suggested these medications were not beneficial and were potentially harmful, we collectively decided to discontinue their use.

Following the acquisition by private equity, there was significant pressure from the administrative side of the business to start using these medications again. The hospices' major client base, skilled nursing facilities, insisted on their use due to the challenges of managing dying patients with secretion issues as well as dissatisfaction of their patients' families. Despite explaining to the nursing homes and our own hospice administrators the lack of data and potential for harm, we were instructed to prescribe them regardless. The economic considerations of the hospice and their clients came first, and the needs of their dying patients, second.

The private equity-owned hospice prioritized maintaining a crucial client relationship with the business — a business that owned several nursing homes in the area, including the ones in question. Unsurprisingly, the very same business also was owned by — you guessed it — another private equity firm. The care of dying patients was simply reduced to a B2B transaction. Patients be damned.

While I wish examples like these were rare, the reality of private equity and venture capital's expanding influence in the American healthcare system is not only undeniable but metastasizing like an uncontrolled malignancy. Instead of providing the much-needed treatment to uproot this cancer, doctors are forced to become the foot soldiers carrying out many of these profit-driven decisions.

This scenario is not novel in our healthcare system, where private physicians and entrepreneurs have long owned specialty hospitals, nursing homes, and dialysis units. The escalating scale and diminished accountability to community well-being, however, are alarming trends.

THE CORPORATE TAKEOVER

In 2021 alone, private equity investors poured over $200 billion into healthcare acquisitions, and over the last decade, their total spending exceeded $1 trillion.[3] Private equity in healthcare refers to the for-profit ownership of healthcare facilities by private parties. Unlike in publicly traded companies, shares of these investor-owned entities are not publicly available and are not subject to the same regulatory requirements. While private equity is not new to our healthcare system, the tactics used by these investors have evolved in destructive ways:

According to the Commonwealth Fund, ownership has shifted from individual physicians or small groups of entrepreneurs to bigger firms that manage funds for wealthy individuals or institutions.[4] These investors lack deep healthcare expertise or a strong ethical commitment to patient care, as illustrated in my hospice example.

The long-term objective tends to be short-term profits. Many firms take out loans on newly acquired acquisitions in order to quickly pay off investors, leaving the healthcare organization to carry the debt.[5] Another profitable but destructive technique is to sell the land, facilities, or other capital assets for a profit and then force the health care organizations to lease them back.

The ultimate aim of these cash-stripping tactics is to flip the asset to a large publicly traded company at a higher valuation than its initial purchase price. To achieve this, they often increase the company's profitability through aggressive cost-cutting measures or by raising prices.

These firms are rapidly acquiring physician practices, especially in high-margin specialties like dermatology. A recent study showed that in 13% of major metropolitan areas, individual private equity firms owned up to half the physician practices in certain specialties.[6]

As a consequence, institutions originally established for the care of the public are being transformed into profit-driven assets, prioritizing revenue generation over their original mission. Physician and healthcare stakeholders who once owned these businesses are being supplanted by revenue-obsessed automatons who favor short-term financial gains over the creation of sustainable enterprises dedicated to serving the very people they were once created for. Margin has overtaken mission.

HIGHER COSTS, WORSE CARE

A stark illustration of this sad state of affairs is the widely publicized bankruptcy of Steward Health System in May 2024. Managed by private equity firm (and corporate raider) Cerberus Capital Management since 2020, the Steward system was floundering and required more than $400 million for recovery. Seeking a swift and painless exit strategy, Cerberus executives convinced the hospital's landlord to provide the necessary funds, allowing them to quickly exit the investment with over $800 million in profit. Meanwhile, Steward was left financially depleted, leading inevitably to a bankruptcy that was all but preordained.[7]

Even without such dramatic bankruptcies, the involvement of private equity often results in a focus on short-term profits and a significant cost escalation. A 2023 study published in the *British Medical Journal* analyzed 55 studies culled from eight countries revealing that healthcare systems newly under private equity ownership experienced harmful cost increases for both patients and payers.[8] The study also raised concerns about the potential impacts on the quality of care.

Further highlighting quality concerns, a 2023 *JAMA* study examined more than 600,000 admissions to hospitals owned by private equity companies and compared them to matched controls.[9] The findings showed a 25.4% increase in hospital-acquired conditions such as falls and line associated blood stream infections. These were in patients who were modestly younger than the controls and assessed to be at lower risk (explaining the original improvement in mortality at 30 days that declined thereafter).

WHY PHYSICIANS ARE SELLING OUT

If it is so evident that private equity is detrimentally affecting healthcare, one might question why dedicated physicians and hospital owners are selling their stakes to these entities, who appear to favor profits over ethical considerations. Why are those of us committed to providing excellent patient care walking away from ownership?

The answer is multifaceted but largely stems from the overwhelming volume and complexity of regulatory compliance imposed by federal and state governments, as well as third-party payers and pharmaceutical companies. For example, a 2017 report from the American Hospital Association pointed out that providers are spending up to $39 billion annually to adhere to administrative requirements related to regulatory compliance.[10] Providers in hospital and post-acute care grapple with 341 and 288 separate regulations respectively in each setting, promulgated by a dizzying list of agencies including the Centers for Medicare & Medicaid Services, the Office of Inspector General, the Office for Civil Rights, and the Office of the National Coordinator for Health Information Technology.

More importantly, it is not just the compliance itself, but the burdensome mechanics of complying. The same study revealed that efforts to meet meaningful use (minimum U.S. government standards for electronic health records) standards impose significant costs on individual providers and hospital systems, yielding minimal financial return or improvement in quality of care.

The IT requirements alone can incur costs amounting to millions for healthcare systems, necessitating regular updates to meet new legislative compliance each year. According to the American Hospital Association, an average-sized community hospital spends approximately $7.6 million annually to uphold compliance with federal regulations.

An egregious example of escalating healthcare compliance is the Health Insurance Portability and Accountability Act (HIPAA). Initially passed in 1996 to facilitate insurance portability when people changed jobs and to protect sensitive health information that could affect future insurability, HIPAA's scope was expanded by the Health Information Technology for Economic and Clinical Health (HITECH) Act in 2019.

This heightened HIPAA's privacy and security rules and increased penalties for violations. As reported by *Medical Economics,* initial estimates predicted compliance costs and personal expenditures to providers to amount to roughly $113 million annually, with ongoing maintenance costs of $14.5 million per year.[11] However, the current annual expense of HIPAA compliance is now estimated to have reached $8.3 billion a year, with each physician bearing an average annual cost of approximately $35,000.

It is understandable, then, why physicians feel forced to sell their practices. The American Medical Association has identified that medical practices require increased reimbursement rates to remain financially viable.[12] Left to their own devices, they neither have the leverage to negotiate better rates with insurers nor to manage the increasingly burdensome costs of escalating government compliance. They find themselves compelled to sell to the highest bidder — often private equity and venture capital firms are the lucky buyers.

HOW PRIVATE EQUITY GETS AROUND COMPLIANCE

While it is true that private equity shares the same burden of costly and time-consuming compliance requirements in today's healthcare environment, their reliance on economies of scale as well as a take-no-prisoners attitude often mitigates these costs' impact on the bottom line. In fact, many larger private equity groups prioritize profitability over adhering to rules designed to safeguard patient privacy and safety, choosing to pay fines instead.

As noted previously, according to *Kaiser Health News,* companies owned or managed by private equity firms have settled at least 34 lawsuits under the False Claims Act, resulting in fines exceeding $500 million from 2014 to 2022.[2] These violations have been so egregious that in March 2024, the Biden administration announced the launch of a comprehensive multiagency effort involving the Federal Trade Commission, the Department of Justice's Antitrust Division, and the U.S. Department of Health and Human Services to scrutinize information regarding private equity practices in healthcare.[13]

Fiduciary versus Standard of Care

Traditionally, the corporate practice of medicine doctrine enforced a commonsense principle that restricted the provision of medical care to all but licensed medical practitioners.[15] This meant that corporations could not obtain medical licenses or directly engage in patient care. Over time, this doctrine has largely faded away as corporate entities began to acquire hospitals and medical practices, although it still holds sway in a few states where enforcement varies. As the corporate practice of medicine doctrine dwindles into obsolescence, it becomes crucial to scrutinize how corporations are shaping medical care, and, more importantly, to whom they are accountable.

Private equity firms take their fiduciary responsibility to shareholders and investors seriously, prioritizing returns and maximizing profits. Conversely, physicians are held to legal standards of care based on accepted medical practice, as well as ethical standards rooted in time-tested oaths such as the Hippocratic Oath. Unfortunately, there is no codified integration of these principles when it comes to the general care of patients by these corporate entities. Doctors, patients, and administrators all have different priorities.

As Laura O. Karas notes in the *Systemic Justice Journal*, there are no specific rules nor ethical obligations that place patients before profits:[14]

> *"In the bliss of this logical disjunctive, corporations have free rein to operate within a system based exclusively on shareholder primacy, with no consideration for the key stakeholder in health care: patients."*

One can only imagine the perverse incentives this disjunction creates. In fact, one doesn't have to speculate at all. It manifests as understaffed nursing homes and hospital floors, overburdened doctors seeing new patients every 10 minutes, and hospice administrators dictating end-of-life treatments based on the needs of the business rather than patient-centered comfort-care.

This scenario paints a healthcare landscape where third parties, in the form of private equity, rapidly acquire healthcare assets, extract profits, and often drive them toward financial distress upon exit. The result is a healthcare system marked by poorer outcomes and escalating costs of care.

ARE DOCTORS TO BLAME?

While it is true that government-induced compliance has eroded physicians' ability to independently run practices and hospitals, does this necessitate transferring ownership to private equity? One could argue that maybe, despite being less financially rewarding, physicians could unite to establish more sustainable systems or, at least, sell to other physician-led groups better equipped to handle the administrative burden.

Unfortunately, non-private equity-based options are often not as viable or even available to struggling physicians trying to stay afloat in an ever-changing sea of tumultous regulations. For various reasons, private equity appears to offer the most practical solutions to physician entrepreneurs within the constrained healthcare environment that has formed around them. According to a 2023 article in *Medical Economics,* several factors make private equity particularly appealing:[15]

- Declining reimbursements from both Medicare and commercial payers.
- Increasing adoption of value-based reimbursement programs becoming the norm like bundled payment initiatives, risk-based reimbursement, and population health.
- Newer reimbursement models requiring a substantial investment in electronic medical records, and data analytics capabilities.
- Intense competition from mega-specialty practices backed by cost-conscious private equity, and retail giants like Walmart and CVS entering the healthcare arena.
- The use of clinical practice as a loss leader by these large conglomerates meant to entice customers to purchase their more lucrative products and services.

The article elaborates that, in the face of these formidable challenges, private equity provides practices with much-needed access to capital, MBA-trained administrators with knowledge of how healthcare systems operate, economies of scale, and the ability to compete with newer and larger players entering the field.

In many respects, these large corporate-based entities provide the most feasible path for practices to survive in a constantly shifting and unpredictable environment. Many physicians prefer to practice under less-than-ideal conditions rather than quit altogether. They feel a responsibility to sustain the viability of the practice for both physicians and non-physician employees alike.

Sadly, the experience of physicians once involved with these private entities often proves disappointing. A study in *JAMA Internal Medicine*, surveying 525 physicians, revealed that 61% viewed private equity's involvement in healthcare negatively while another 28.8% had a neutral opinion.[16] Among the 29 respondents who had experience working directly for private equity, only 44.8% expressed interest in remaining with their employer compared to 77.8% of those working in other practice settings.

Ultimately, physicians feel powerless in maintaining their own practices and yet trapped after working for private equity. This sense of powerlessness permeates the doctor-patient relationship, as physicians become the face of corporate decision-making such as patient volume, formulary decisions, and staffing requirements.

A recent study conducted by NORC at The University of Chicago surveyed 1,000 physicians employed by hospitals or health systems, venture capital or private equity firms, health insurance companies or subsidiaries, or staffing agencies from July 17 to August 7, 2023. The aim was to gauge the impact of ownership changes on their experiences.[17] The survey revealed that nearly 60% of physicians identified the loss of autonomy as a significant issue adversely affecting the doctor-patient relationship. They cited insufficient time, breakdowns in communication, fragmented care coordination, deprioritization of patients' needs and autonomy, and limitations on patient choice as major barriers to effective patient-provider relationships.

TOWARD BUILDING A BETTER SYSTEM

To suggest private equity should be entirely removed from our healthcare system would be, to say the least, misguided. At their best, these companies can inject substantial capital, foster innovation, achieve cost-savings and efficiency, and enhance the effectiveness of what is acknowledged to be a somewhat flawed system. They have the potential to revitalize struggling physician practices and leverage economies of scale to help navigate the complex web of compliance that burdens private practitioners. For this positive potential to be realized on a broader scale, however, several crucial steps need to be taken.

Better Regulation

In March 2024, the Federal Trade Commission, the Department of Justice's Antitrust Division, and the U.S. Department of Health and Human Services launched a public inquiry seeking a request for information regarding the role of private equity-backed transactions in healthcare. FTC Chair Lina Khan pointed out three deeply concerning "extractive" practices:[18]

- Short-term, low-risk flip and strip approaches.
- Concentration strategies (roll-ups) that consolidate market power and weaken competition.
- Acquisitions of competing firms within the same sector, potentially reducing market diversity and consumer choice.

As Khan noted:[18]

> *"A common theme across comments is that growing financialization in the health care industry can force medical professionals to subordinate their own medical judgement to corporate decision-makers' profit motives at the expense of patient health."*

Aligning Fiduciary Standards with Ethical Standards of Care

Physicians are consistently held to rigorous ethical and professional standards of care. Every medical student in the United States learns and pledges some version of an ethical code. Whether it is the Hippocratic Oath or the Declaration of Geneva, all physicians are sworn to protect and serve their patients, fellow colleagues, and society. Additionally, our profession is governed by standards of care set by state and federal regulatory bodies, medical societies, and America's strikingly punitive medicolegal system.

Private equity and venture capital firms involved in healthcare must be held to these same high standards. While various organizations have begun to codify ethical practices for the business of healthcare, these standards have not been universally mandated nor widely adopted. Examples include the National Association of Healthcare Quality's (NAHQ) code of ethics and conduct[19] and the American College of Healthcare Executives (ACHE) code of ethics.[20]

These documents should not only define expected behaviors for individual healthcare executives in complex decision-making roles, but also outline a vision for how ethical for-profit healthcare institutions behave in general, and in regard to the well-being of the public in particular. In healthcare, unlike other sectors, financial gains must come secondary to ensuring not only the safety of our patients, but also the diligent stewardship of public funds collected for the greater good.

Healthcare funding was never intended to enrich business tycoons; its purpose is to deliver this deeply important service to our people.

Durable Consequences

One reason private equity has been able to circumvent healthcare regulation effectively is that the penalties imposed for improper behavior are not sufficiently economically impactful to deter misconduct. Imposing million-dollar fines on companies that stand to make billions is insufficient to discourage predatory behavior. For example, in 2011, Small Smiles, owned by FORBA Holdings LLC, incurred a $24 million fine under the False Claims Act for delivering unnecessary care.[21]

While a $24 million penalty may sound substantial at first, it pales in comparison to the $161 million in revenues Small Smiles collected from Medicaid and New York's Children's Health Insurance Program (CHIP) that very same year.[22] Moreover, FORBA filed for bankruptcy in 2012, restructured, and maddeningly continued operations, suggesting that the penalty did little to change its operations. Predictably, a few years later, after failing to mend its ways, Small Smiles faced bankruptcy again in 2015 after being forced by the government into a settlement of $39 million.[23]

If penalties fail to significantly affect financial operations, lasting and enduring behavioral change is unlikely to occur.

Bring Back Private Practice

There is compelling evidence that small private practices still deliver care that is superior to or at least on par with that of large private equity-based practices.[24] The primary challenge lies in the escalating overhead costs, intense competition, and the crush of burdensome compliance requirements that threaten the viability of private practices.

Logic dictates, however, that a decentralized system inherently avoids leveraging market dominance for profit extraction. Unlike our current corporate overlords, physicians are guided by ethical guidelines stemming from professional oaths taken seriously enough to be a consistent part of the medical initiation process over the centuries. Furthermore, they are legally bound by standards of care that prioritize the primacy of patient-centered care — constraints absent in private equity models.

Why should we allow these third parties to siphon wealth from the system without enhancing tangible benefits in quality of care?

To preserve private practice in the American healthcare system, we must ease the vice grip of governmental compliance, meaningful use, and third-party regulations like prior authorization. It is only when we allow doctors to spend their time doctoring, that we will truly create a patient-centered medical system.

The financial and organizational burden of administrative minutia is driving our healthcare dollars right into the hands of those who are ready and able to exploit the system. We are disempowering the main stakeholders, healthcare providers and patients, in favor of profit-driven third parties. We must stop.

• • • • • •

Medicine is not the only field in which corporate America has, at times, overstepped its boundaries, prioritizing profits over people. We have a storied history of allowing businesses to exert unchecked influence over the welfare of our workers, consumers, and paychecks, only to be regulated by protective legislation in due course.

These discussions prompt us to define our nation's approach to capitalism, weigh the merits and risks of socialism, and legislate the balance between corporate interests and individual rights. This ongoing struggle is as old as our country itself and has unfolded numerous times throughout our history. And a major weapon in this battle, as Upton Sinclair demonstrated at the turn of the 20th century, is the power of storytelling.

The Jungle/Upton Sinclair

The Jungle, by Upton Sinclair, became an instant sensation upon it release in 1906.[25] As a committed socialist, Sinclair aimed to expose the harsh conditions endured by Chicago's meatpacking workers at the turn of the century. *The Jungle*, meant to be a metaphor for capitalism, depicted, through vivid and often graphic images such as blood and guts strewn across the walls of an unsanitary work environment, the atrocities suffered by powerless and poorly paid employees.

Although Sinclair's primary intention was to advocate for labor rights, the popularity of his novel unexpectedly spurred a national outcry, and eventually legislation, to improve the quality and safety of food manufacturing. In direct response to Sinclair's novel, Teddy Roosevelt signed the first comprehensive federal food safety laws on June 30, 1906.

Despite Sinclair's disappointment that his initial goals for labor reform were overshadowed by the food safety movement, many credit his work with the rise of labor unions and the eventual passage of the National Labor Relations Act (NLRA) of 1935.

The NLRA, among other things, encourages collective bargaining by protecting workers' full freedom of association. Furthermore, it provides employees at private workplaces the right to seek better working conditions without fear of retaliation.[26]

Sinclair's powerful storytelling shows how literature can provoke profound societal change, even revolution, when challenging entrenched and powerful private interests and paving the way for reform and progress.

PART TWO.

How Your Doctor Became a Pawn

ON AUGUST 29, 2005 AT 6:10 A.M., one of the deadliest natural disasters in history struck the city of New Orleans, Louisiana. The city would suffer most of its devastation in the days following the aftermath of the initial impact as the deadly toll became clear. Just six hours after Hurricane Katrina touched down, at 2:00 p.m., 53 levees breached, allowing water from Lake Pontchartrain and the Gulf of Mexico to flow into the city. New Orleans was under water.

Approximately seven miles from the breached canals stood the Memorial Medical Center in Uptown New Orleans. The hurricane and resultant storm knocked out the hospital's power and water supply, pushing temperatures inside above 100 degrees.[1] The beleaguered staff, severely undermanned and fatigued after more than two days on duty, worked tirelessly to evacuate, triage, and care for the critically ill patients who were unable to be evacuated. Then, as recounted by *The New York Times Magazine*, the unimaginable happened:[2]

> *"At about 2 a.m. on Wednesday, Aug. 31 — nearly 48 hours after Katrina made landfall near New Orleans — Memorial's backup generators sputtered and stopped. Ewing Cook later described the sudden silence as the "sickest sound" of his life. In LifeCare on the seventh floor, critically ill patients began suffering the consequences. Alarm bells clanged as life-support monitors and ventilators*

> *switched to brief battery reserves while continuing to force air into the lungs of seven patients. In about a half-hour, the batteries failed and the regular hiss of mechanical breaths ceased."*

Faced with overwhelming fatigue, suffering patients, and a dearth of outside assistance, Memorial staff, including an oncological surgeon named Dr. Anna Pou, made the heartbreaking decision to administer a combination of morphine and versed to a number of critically ill patients. These patients were too frail to move to safety, suffering greatly, or were unlikely to survive the impending hardships. Subsequently, these patients died swiftly and peacefully.

In July 2006, nearly a year after Hurricane Katrina, Dr. Pou, alongside two Memorial Medical Center nurses, were arrested and faced charges of second-degree murder in connection with the deaths of four patients during the Katrina crisis.[3] A grand jury, however, refused to indict Pou for murder, and all charges against her were dismissed in July 2007.

Since then, Dr. Pou has successfully advocated for three laws in Louisiana granting immunity to healthcare professionals from most civil lawsuits arising from their actions during disasters. While ethical debates persist regarding her decisions, Dr. Pou's case serves as a stark illustration of the challenges and ethical dilemmas clinicians face in extreme circumstances. What many people outside the medical profession often overlook is that every decision involving life and death, whether in the midst of a natural disaster or in routine medical practice, is inherently critical.

Anna Pou, like many physicians, confronted split-second, life-altering decisions. Her actions were profoundly influenced by the inadequate resources provided by the hospital and the for-profit private company that owned the long-term nursing floor where many of the patients were euthanized. Subsequently, she faced not only public scrutiny but also legal repercussions from faltering governmental bodies that shared responsibility for the lack of resources during the disaster.

Dr. Anna Pou became a pawn of the system. Your doctor is no different.

As explored in Chapter One, patients often perceive doctors as major players in the current challenges plaguing our healthcare system today. However, upon closer examination, it becomes evident that healthcare providers themselves have also become leverage in a system that no longer supports them.

Third parties have employed a divide-and-conquer strategy, fostering discord among the primary stakeholders in our healthcare system. This intentionally orchestrated chaos allows these entities to exploit the system while we remain preoccupied with internal disagreements. Deliberate efforts have fractured the doctor-patient relationship. Inadvertently, we have allowed ourselves to be mischaracterized as agents of those pulling the strings, rather than recognizing our shared vulnerability as mere puppets in this complex scenario.

Part Two of this book will delve into how doctors, much like patients, have been manipulated — this time by the medicolegal industrial complex, electronic medical records companies, and even the government. We find ourselves allies with our patients in a struggle that either innocently goes unrecognized or more sinisterly unacknowledged.

And regrettably, we are losing this battle.

CHAPTER FIVE.

Your Doctor Is also Struggling (The Doctor's View)

FOR YEARS, I WROTE A BLOG titled *In My Humble Opinion,* sharing insights into the life of a doctor. I filled the pages with stories about patient care and the struggles of those behind the stethoscope. Over time, as my blog gained popularity, I started receiving feedback from a few of my patients who stumbled upon my online writing.

One particular afternoon stands out vividly from all those years of writing my blog. Jacob, a patient with whom I had built a long-standing relationship filled with pleasant visits, light moments, and camaraderie, came in for a routine blood pressure check. That specific afternoon, however, his demeanor was notably somber as he entered my office.

With genuine concern, I gently inquired about his well-being and the reason for his visit. Jacob, to my great surprise, placed his hand on my shoulder, looked me directly in the eyes, and asked how I was doing. For what felt like a long moment we simply held each other's gaze, silently connecting in a way that transcended our usual doctor-patient dynamic.

Little did I know, Jacob was a long-time reader of my blog and was deeply moved by a recent post where I shared my experience of losing a long-time patient. It was a perspective he had never considered before — suddenly, he began to reflect not just on his own health, but on the well-being of his doctors. As he later confided to me, he had always taken our presence for granted, never realizing the challenges we faced in caring for him.

That day marked a profound shift in our relationship. We evolved from doctor and patient to partners in the ongoing struggle for his health and mine. That partnership endured many twists and turns over the years: his cancer diagnosis, my transition between medical systems, the devastating loss of his wife, and the joys of my children's births.

The magic in our transformed relationship lay in the mutual realization that we were allies. While caregivers have long recognized (albeit imperfectly) the battles faced by patients, Jacob's newfound empathy for my struggles as a physician created a genuine sense of reciprocity between us.

It is a reciprocity that I, as a physician, aim to illustrate in this chapter — a reciprocity hindered primarily by a lack of trust. This lack of trust between doctors and patients often arises from concerns about three main issues: fears surrounding competence (malpractice), access (time), and incentives (money). The ultimate consequence, for many physicians, is burnout.

Most patients are surprised that their doctors are struggling in today's healthcare environment and have become victims to some of the very same destructive forces they have. Doctors and patients share more common ground than either party realizes, especially in how they contribute to enriching others' lives.

Let's take a look at how third parties frame these issues to the detriment of physicians and further exploit the doctor-patient relationship, resulting in losses for both parties.

QUESTIONABLE COMPETENCE

While we will explore the malpractice crisis extensively in Chapter Six, it's crucial to acknowledge here the extent and pervasiveness of the problem. As I mentioned in the Introduction to this book, my decision to leave medicine was precipitated by being named in a malpractice lawsuit — an ordeal that spanned years, incurred substantial financial costs, and profoundly shook my confidence and mental well-being. Even though I was eventually exonerated and dismissed from the suit, the emotional and professional impact was lasting.

I am not alone in this experience.

According to a study by the American Medical Association, nearly a third of practicing physicians had reported being sued as of 2022.[1] This analysis underscores that for most physicians, it is not a matter of if, but when. When age is taken into account, the likelihood of physicians being sued increases to 46.8% by the time they reach the age of 54. These statistics vary significantly by specialty, with low-risk fields like allergy immunology facing lawsuits as low as 7%, while high-risk, procedure-oriented specialties like obstetrics can see rates as high as 62%. Interestingly, women tend to face lower liability risks compared to men.

The repercussions of such litigation have enduring effects that often go unnoticed by the public, affecting a physician's mental well-being and the quality of care delivered. Research indicates that more than half of physicians experience significant psychological distress following a malpractice claim.[2] Equally concerning, nearly half of the respondents (45.39%) reported making practice changes, such as viewing patients as potential plaintiffs (45.39%), undergoing medicolegal training (37.94%), ordering additional tests more liberally (36.17%), and avoiding certain types of high-risk patients (21.63%) and procedures (19.85%).

Physicians are deeply dissatisfied with the impact of the medicolegal environment but feel helpless to effect change. A 2011 study published in the *Archives of Internal Medicine* sheds light on this sense of helplessness, revealing that 42% of nationally surveyed doctors believed that their patients were receiving "too much medicine," with 76% saying that fears of malpractice were the main driver of aggressive and expensive care.[3] Additionally, 40% attributed over-testing to having insufficient time to spend with each patient.

In this noxious environment, no one emerges victorious except perhaps malpractice attorneys. The doctor-patient relationship is marred by distrust, with physicians viewing every patient through the lens of becoming a potential litigant. And even more disturbing, patients in urgent need of medical attention are sometimes avoided due to the complexities involved in their care. Moreover, these factors contribute to the rising costs of healthcare, a topic we will explore in detail in the next chapter. This includes the expense incurred from ordering additional and sometimes unnecessary tests to mitigate liability concerns.

LIMITED ACCESS TO CARE

The practice of medicine today is a herculean undertaking for several reasons. Firstly, a rise in compliance and administrative tasks have largely fallen on the shoulders of busy physicians. According to a 2014 article in the *International Journal of Health Services,* average U.S. physicians dedicated one-sixth of their time to administrative duties, a figure that has significantly increased since the introduction of electronic medical records.[4] By 2018, this burden had increased to nearly 20 hours per week, as reported by a Medscape Physician Compensation study.[5]

Secondly, the "guidelineification" of medical practice has resulted in an expanding array of tasks and responsibilities, particularly in relation to general medical care. This responsibility is increasingly borne by a cadre of beleaguered primary care physicians. A simulation study conducted by the University of Chicago in August 2022 revealed that primary care doctors would require an average of 27 hours per day to meet all guidelines-based care expectations.[6] This includes 14.1 hours daily for preventive care, 7.2 hours for chronic disease care, 2.2 hours for acute care, and 3.2 hours for documentation and inbox management.

And of course, these calculations highlighting the overwhelming demands placed on physicians, don't even allow time for a bathroom break or a few minutes to eat lunch!

We simply are not training enough physicians to meet these demands. A 2024 study by the Association of American Medical Colleges projected that the United States will face a physician shortage of up to 86,000 physicians by 2036.[7] The study also highlighted some concerning demographic trends:

- The U.S. population is projected to grow by 8.4%.
- The population aged 65 and older is projected to grow by 34.1%.
- There will be a 54.7% rise in the population aged 75 and older.
- Physicians aged 65 or older make up 20% of the clinical physician workforce.

We are heading toward a disaster!

Furthermore, in what has been dubbed medicine's great resignation, physicians are leaving their jobs at an unprecedented rate. A 2021 study published in the *Mayo Clinic Proceedings* indicated that one in four physicians was likely to leave their job within the next two years.[8] Even more concerning, one in three planned to reduce their work hours in the next 12 months.

The combination of these factors is resulting in a severe lack of access to care in the United States, particularly in terms of primary care physicians. According to the Kaiser Family Foundation, more than 100 million people currently lack adequate access to primary care, a number that has doubled since 2014.[9] The percentage of primary care doctors for adults has been declining rapidly toward the 25% mark, posing a threat to Americans' ability to access essential care.[10]

The consequences couldn't be more dire. As outlined by the Office of Disease Prevention and Health Promotion in their literature summary for their Healthy People 2030 initiative, a lack of primary care access:[11]

- May increase the risk of poor health outcomes and health disparities broadly.
- May lead individuals to delay or forgo needed care.
- May mean that uninsured adults are less likely to receive preventive services for chronic conditions such as diabetes, cancer, and cardiovascular disease.

Another emerging issue is that when access to low-cost primary care is limited, frustrated patients resort to more expensive options, such as utilizing emergency rooms for non-emergency needs. The financial burden on our healthcare system due to these practices has been estimated to reach as high as $47 billion annually.[12]

INCENTIVES

The erosion of trust between doctors and patients is particularly evident and fraught with consequences when it comes to incentives. Historically, physicians have seldom been incentivized to deny care or protect money earmarked for medical treatment. The thrust of our healthcare system, however, has been to create a new class of highly educated gatekeepers who occasionally are tasked to do just that.

This transformation can be traced back to the Health Maintenance Organization Act of 1973, which established the legal framework for modern day health maintenance organizations (HMOs).[13] The primary objective was to ensure patients received appropriate care and referrals by designating the primary care physicians as gatekeepers who oversee and manage care comprehensively and act as intermediaries between the patient and healthcare specialists. It became their responsibility to determine the necessity of referrals and procedures.

This arrangement creates an ethical conundrum. Physicians are not only charged with providing optimal clinical care to each individual patient, but also with responsibly managing the nation's finite healthcare resources. Predictably, this dual role can lead to conflicts, especially in a population sensitive to the notion of healthcare rationing.

Research from the *British Medical Journal* explored the impact of the gatekeeping model on the National Health Service.[14] Their findings reveal the complicated effects of such models: While healthcare costs decreased and utilization was managed, patient satisfaction and survival rates among cancer patients were lower. Even if gatekeeping demonstrates equivalent quality care, it tends to foster a confrontational or paternalistic relationship between doctors and patients.

Regrettably, this dynamic is further influenced by the next generation of gatekeeping models known as pay-for-performance or value-based purchasing. In these models, physicians receive higher compensation based on meeting specific quality benchmarks or sometimes overall cost savings. In the United States, such models gained prominence in the early 2000s with the advent of accountable care organizations or ACOs, aimed at addressing both healthcare cost and improving care quality.[15]

Defined by the American Academy of Family Physicians, an ACO is a consortium of healthcare providers who collectively assume responsibility for the quality, cost, and coordination of care, with aligned incentives for a specific patient population.[16] These ACOs once again position physicians as guardians of the financial health of the nation, often requiring them to make difficult decisions, including the potential denial of care for individuals in the interest of societal benefit. For example, imagine a situation where a costly treatment is declined for a patient due to its 10% chance of success. While a doctor advocating solely for the patient might opt for this treatment, the same doctor, acting as a gatekeeper within an ACO, should determine that the expense is unjustifiable for the broader population. Who should our doctors serve?

I know my answer to this question.

While ACOs have faced scrutiny regarding their ability to fulfill promises of enhanced care quality, there is a recognized risk, as highlighted in an *NEJM Catalyst* article, that pay-for-performance systems diminish clinician job satisfaction and intrinsic motivation.[17] Moreover, these systems can divert time and attention away from aspects of care that are truly essential, focusing instead on metrics that are easier to measure.

In either case, these systems increasingly position physicians as controllers of the purse strings of our healthcare system, tasks for which they were neither trained nor inclined to perform. The result, as with so many forces in healthcare today, is burnout — an epidemic that pervades the practice of medicine.

PHYSICIAN BURNOUT

Burnout has become increasingly prevalent among healthcare practitioners, a trend exacerbated by COVID-19. According to the most recent data from a national burnout survey series by the American Medical Association, by the end of 2021, 63% of physicians reported experiencing symptoms of burnout, a significant increase from 38% in 2020.[18]

There has been a long-standing debate over whether the generalized fatigue experienced in medicine should be labeled as burnout or characterized differently. Defined by the World Health Organization, burnout encompasses three dimensions:[19]

- Feelings of energy depletion or exhaustion.
- Increased mental distance from one's job or feelings of negativism or cynicism related to one's job.
- Reduced professional efficacy.

However, many in the medical field argue that what healthcare practitioners are truly grappling with is more accurately described as moral injury. In a 2018 article, Simon Talbot and Wendy Dean highlight that attributing these challenges solely to burnout implies a lack of resourcefulness or resilience.[20] They propose a different interpretation of what is really happening:[21]

> *"Moral injury occurs when we perpetrate, bear witness to, or fail to prevent an act that transgresses our deeply held moral beliefs. In the health care context, that deeply held moral belief is the oath each of us took when embarking on our paths as health care providers: Put the needs of patients first. That oath is the lynchpin of our working lives and our guiding principle when searching for the right course*

of action. But as clinicians, we are increasingly forced to consider the demands of other stakeholders — the electronic medical record (EMR), the insurers, the hospital, the health care system, even our own financial security — before the needs of our patients. Every time we are forced to make a decision that contravenes our patients' best interests, we feel a sting of moral injustice. Over time, these repetitive insults amass into moral injury."

This third-party interference lies at the heart of moral injury, driving a wedge between doctors and patients while disconnecting healthcare costs from the actual services provided. It's undeniable that the entire population bears the burden. As this chapter draws to a close, it's crucial to acknowledge that this burden is equally borne by our nation's caregivers: doctors, nurses, social workers, physical therapists, occupational therapists, chaplains, nurse practitioners, certified nursing assistants... we are all paying the price.

• • • • • •

The most harrowing night of my life occurred over two decades ago in an ICU. As a resident physician, I found myself alone with the hospital's most critically ill patients and suffered through the death of an elderly man as I struggled to provide lifesaving care for which I had not yet received sufficient training. That night marked the beginning of a decade-long descent into burnout (or moral injury if you prefer) fueled by the relentless demands of patient care, the specter of malpractice, an overwhelming administrative workload, and a loss of autonomy over the type of medicine I aspired to practice.

A court summons to defend my medical decisions in an unrelated case many years later coupled with the sheer lack of financial stability prompted a solemn vow to leave medicine behind. I hoped to escape the profound sense of moral injury that had been plaguing me.

Unfortunately, my experience is not unique among clinicians in our medical system. For some, it's the constant fear of malpractice. For others, it's the anguish of feeling inadequately trained or the guilt of not being able to save a patient. Many struggle with the weight of medical debt and the desire to leave a profession that no longer fulfills them.

Sometimes, the outcome is far more tragic than just loss of professional autonomy or job dissatisfaction. Each year, 300-400 physicians tragically take their own lives.[22] Medical students experience rates of depression that are 15%-30% higher than the general population. In 2019, on an episode of the *Earn & Invest* podcast, I had the pleasure of interviewing Robyn Symon, whose documentary "Do No Harm" sheds light on the profound struggles faced by physicians in training.

Do No Harm: Exposing the Hippocratic Hoax/ Robyn Symon

"Jumping off hospital rooftops, hanging themselves in janitorial closets, overdosing on drugs — they're A students and their suicides are often like well-planned school projects. Doctors are our healers, yet they have the highest rate of suicide among any profession. Medical students and families of physicians touched by suicide come out of the shadows to expose this silent epidemic and the truth about a sick healthcare system that not only drives our brilliant young doctors to take their own lives but puts patients lives at risk too."

In this pointed documentary, Robyn Symon, two-time Emmy Award winner, follows Hawkins Mecham, a fourth-year medical student who survived a suicide attempt the previous year.[23] Mecham joins forces with John and Michele Dietl, parents who turn their grief into advocacy after their son, Kevin, tragically took his own life just three months shy of graduating medical school. Together, they push for legislation requiring medical schools to report depression levels — a crucial first step in addressing and resolving the pervasive suicide crisis among medical professionals.

Symon uses these compelling true-life characters to explore how we got here — how an unhealthy training environment has led to self-harm, bullying, assembly line medicine, and a population of overworked and debt-laden trainees. She further follows the money and exposes the exploitation of medical students as a cheap labor force by hospital systems, where residents are forced to work marathon shifts up to 28 hours, risking patient safety.

"Do No Harm," highlighting the advocacy of Dr. Pamela Wible, has significantly raised awareness of physician suicide. In 2022, Congress passed the Lorna Breen Act in response to these efforts, aimed at improving mental health support for physicians. The legislation includes provisions to:[24]

- Establish grants for health professionals to develop evidence-based strategies to reduce burnout and the associated secondary mental health conditions related to job stress.
- Launch a national campaign to encourage health professionals to prioritize their mental health and utilize available mental and behavioral health services.
- Fund grants for employee education and peer-support programming.
- Initiate a comprehensive study on the mental health and burnout of doctors and other health professionals.

Dr. Lorna Breen, the act's namesake, tragically died by suicide in April 2022 after enduring the intense strain of treating COVID-19 patients. Her story, alongside those of Mecham, the Dietls, and countless other physician tragedies each year, underscores the urgent need for systemic change and greater support for medical professionals' mental well-being.

CHAPTER SIX.

Who Defines the Standard of Care? (Competence)

THE LEGAL DEFINITION OF MALPRACTICE hinges on the concept of the standard of care. Simply put, standard of care is what a reasonable physician would do in an identical set of circumstances. Each year in the United States, between 15,000 and 20,000 malpractice suits are filed based on suspected breaches of this standard,[1] resulting in payouts totaling $42 billion from 2010 to 2019 alone.[2]

A fundamental issue within our system arises from the fact that any patient can allege medical malpractice against a physician. According to the American Medical Association, one in three clinicians will be sued at least once during their career,[3] with significantly elevated rates in high-risk specialties, approaching nearly 100%.

So, who determines whether the standard of care has been breached? The final decision unfortunately arrives after many years of pretrial and trial proceedings, significant financial expenditures from all parties, and profound emotional fallout from doctors, patients, and their families alike. Litigation comes at a steep cost.

An AMA Policy Perspectives piece highlighted a troubling statistic: In 2015, 68.2% of all malpractice suits were either dropped, dismissed, or withdrawn, resulting in no compensation for the plaintiff.[4] That's more than two-thirds of cases! Furthermore, physicians prevail in eight of 10 cases that do eventually proceed to trial.[5] Breaches of the standard of care are measurably infrequent.

We're investing substantial time and money litigating cases that ultimately have little chance of succeeding. Why do we continue down this fruitless path?

Before delving more deeply into the statistics and the complex medico-legal system that perpetuates them, I'd like to introduce you to Francine. In her early 70s, chronically ill, and legally blind, Francine became an unwitting and unacknowledged casualty of this system. Hers is a story that cannot be fully understood through data alone.

FRANCINE'S STORY

Every day, Francine said a little prayer for her doctor — sometimes upon awakening, often before drifting off to sleep at night. Her world had narrowed significantly since Simon, her husband, passed away the year before. With no children or close friends, Francine relied heavily on Doctor G to make sure that her needs were met.

Initially, Francine enjoyed visiting the office and chatting with the receptionist. As Francine's mobility declined, however, Doctor G began making house calls. It was not just the physical strain; the lingering depression following Simon's death weighed heavily on her. The antidepressant pills, however, were beginning to take effect. The few colors she could still discern seemed brighter, and there was even talk of her niece visiting from Ohio.

Then came devastating news: Doctor G was retiring from medicine and leaving the practice. Francine had always imagined that because he was much younger than her previous doctor, he would care for her until the end.

Her last visit to the office was bittersweet. Though her physical condition had improved quite a bit, meeting Doctor G's replacement left her feeling disheartened. The new doctor appeared hurried and less warm.

A few days later, as Francine experienced a brief bout of chest pain while watching television in her living room on a brisk Chicago day, she hesitated to call her new doctor. Outside, rooftops glistened with a fresh dusting of snow. Doctor G would have stopped by her apartment on the way out of the office and assessed her condition in the comfort of her own home. But with this new doctor — well, who could say?

As Francine drifted off to sleep, she pondered why such a young doctor would be leaving medicine so prematurely, and who would care for all of his elderly patients in the future. In fact, it was likely her last thought before slipping into unconsciousness. Perhaps she felt a fleeting pain or a moment of breathlessness as the massive heart attack overtook her. We'll never know.

We also will never know if Doctor G would have indeed visited her in the apartment or sent her to the hospital. In any number of alternate realities, she might have received appropriate and timely care and welcomed her niece into town with open arms a week later.

Instead, she died of a broken heart.

A PROMISE TO MYSELF

Early in my medical training, a close friend faced unjust accusations of malpractice, enduring a grueling trial marked by self-doubt and eventual vindication. Witnessing her ordeal, I made a solemn vow to myself: If ever sued, guilty or not, justified or not, I would leave medicine without hesitation. The trauma of standing trial would destroy the will to practice medicine again.

The unspoken reality of being named in a lawsuit fundamentally alters how one practices the delicate art of medicine. Objectivity is lost, replaced by an instinct to overcorrect and protect oneself. The focus shifts from delivering the best care for the patient, to avoiding the trauma of being sued again. We become paranoid and overcautious.

The shift is supported by the data. A 2018 study from the National Bureau of Economic Research revealed that doctors' fear of lawsuits increases the intensity and cost of hospital care by 5%, without yielding measurably better outcomes.[6]

In my case, supposition became chilling reality one cold winter night when, at my front door I was handed a summons to appear before a judge, while my wife and children sat quietly watching television in the adjacent family room. What ensued was a calamity spanning four years, costing my insurance company and me thousands of dollars in missed work and deductibles, ultimately leading to my departure from private practice and clinical medicine altogether.

The conclusion of the story was rather anticlimactic. After years of turmoil, I was dropped from the lawsuit when my deposition testimony finally persuaded the nursing home involved to settle with the deceased patient's family.

I received my own personal reprieve a few months earlier, before the settlement, when the plaintiffs' attorney openly confessed in court to the judge that he had never intended to pursue the complaint against me. He had used my testimony as leverage to extract a larger settlement from the nursing home and hospital.

I was a connecting puzzle piece. A pawn. A resource to be exploited in the attorney's high-stakes blame game. The attorney sensed that the roulette wheel of fate was poised to yield a significant payout.

The attorney positioned himself as an advocate for the patient and their family, but everyone involved understood the reality. The nursing home had committed no wrongdoing — an indisputable truth acknowledged by all parties. Economically, settling made more sense than proceeding to court regardless of the outcome — win or lose. The nursing home's attorney, wise to the financial realities, recognized that prevailing in a protracted legal battle would exceed the costs of a settlement.

For the patient's family, the settlement provided only modest compensation when compared to the years of anguish and extended grief caused by contentious litigation. No amount of money could replace their loved one. The past could not be undone.

Meanwhile, the plaintiff's attorney walked away with a substantial percentage of the settlement. In fact, he was the only one smiling at the end of this heartbreaking fiasco.

THE SPOILS OF WAR

By the way, I am Doctor G. Francine was one of my patients. My decision to leave medicine undoubtedly contributed to her premature death, as well as that of several other patients who passed away shortly after I closed my practice. It wasn't just Francine. There was George, battling brittle diabetes for years who was just barely hanging on before I left, and Sasha, prone to congestive heart failure exacerbations when she travelled out of town. Her new doctor, unfamiliar with her medical history, took a more lenient approach to her restrictions, not having been involved in her last hospital admission.

When doctors leave their practices, they take with them invaluable knowledge and expertise accumulated over years of caring for their patients — most of which has never been formally written down. This issue has been exacerbated even further in this post-pandemic era. According to a 2022 report by *Definitive Healthcare,* 334,000 healthcare providers exited the workforce in 2021, including 117,000 doctors.[7] The primary care specialties suffered especially significant losses, with internal medicine seeing a departure of 15,000 MDs and family practice losing 13,000 practitioners.

Patients aren't the only ones affected. When I left my practice, the livelihoods of my staff — secretaries, lab techs, and others — were also impacted. Physicians often drive the revenue for medical offices, and without their presence, the financial resources to cover salaries and essential services dwindle.

Attributing the entire "great resignation" and physician shortage solely to the malpractice crisis would be premature. However, it's undeniable that concerns and anxieties related to malpractice contribute significantly to burnout and frustration among physicians. In fact, psychiatrists recently coined the term "medical malpractice stress syndrome" or MMSS to describe the traumatic aftermath physicians endure following malpractice lawsuits.[8] Those affected by MMSS often suffer through isolation, helplessness, and hopelessness, which can increase the risk of depression and even suicide.

It also is a primary driver in the decision to leave medicine.

THE CULPABILITY MYTH

The culpability myth has become pervasive in society today. Attributing the shortcomings of our healthcare system primarily to the mistakes of healthcare providers has played a pivotal role in undermining the doctor-patient relationship. While the Institute of Medicine's report *To Err is Human* aimed not to blame compassionate healthcare professionals but rather to critique systems of care, its consequences have inadvertently shifted blame on to individual caregivers.

Google the phrase "how common is medical malpractice?" and you will find countless results from plaintiff's law firms in every nook and cranny of the United States. Their claims echo *To Err is Human* and the innumerable follow-up studies. They proclaim:

- Medical errors rank as the third leading cause of death in the United States.
- 400,000 people succumb to medical errors each year.
- 10% of all deaths in the United States stem from of medical errors.
- Medical mistakes are prevalent enough to rank as one of the top causes of death each year.

The rhetoric is rife, yet none of these statistics can justify why two-thirds of malpractice suits are eventually dropped or why 80% of cases that go to trial find that there was no breach in the standard of care. The presumption is that medical malpractice, when scrutinized under the microscope of actual evidence, is far less widespread than previously believed. This assertion is backed by an article from McGill University titled "Medical Error Is Not the Third Leading Cause of Death," which critiques both *To Err Is Human* and the 2016 *British Medical Journal* article that proposed the one-third estimate.[8] The McGill article argues that these estimates were significantly flawed due to errors in extrapolating from limited data sets. In the authors' own words:[9]

> *"What we end up with, when we look beyond the scary headline of medical errors as the third leading cause of death, is an analysis of studies that were never meant to look at deaths caused by medical errors, often reporting a very small number of deaths from populations that are not generalizable to the whole of the United States, and being combined in a crude way. The BMJ's higher estimate of preventable deaths due to medical error — 440,000 patients a year — translates to 62% of all hospital deaths, as was pointed out by Drs. Benjamin L. Mazer and Chadi Nabhan. That nearly two thirds of all deaths occurring in hospitals would be due to medical error strains credulity."*

The resultant zeitgeist completely overlooks that our medical system is plagued by systems-based errors exacerbated by excessive interference from the very third parties benefitting from this confusion and chaos. The overly complex medicolegal environment directly encourages defensive over-documentation, unnecessary lab testing, and the reluctance of cautious physicians to treat high-risk patients.

These distractions place physicians and nurses squarely in front of computer screens rather than at the bedside. They clutter our brains with subjective concerns about liability instead of focusing on objective patient care, ultimately increasing, not reducing, the overall risk of malpractice.

And everyone loses. Or at least almost everyone.

WHO ARE THE WINNERS

Table 3, from a 2010 *Health Affairs* article, outlines the estimated national costs of our medical liability system for the year 2008.[10] The numbers in

Estimates Of National Costs Of The Medical Liability System

Indemnity payments	$5.72	Good as to the total; moderate as to the precision of the split among the components
Economic damages	$3.15	
Noneconomic damages	$2.40	
Punitive damages	$0.17	
Administrative expenses	$4.13[a]	Moderate
Plaintiff legal expenses	$2.00[b]	Good
Defendant legal expenses	$1.09	Moderate
Other overhead expenses	$3.04	Good
Defensive medicine costs	$45.59	Low
Hospital services	$38.79	
Physician/clinical services	$6.80	
Other costs		
Lost clinician work time	$0.20	Moderate
Price effects	—[b]	Low
Reputational/emotional harm	—[b]	No evidence
Total	$55.64	

TABLE 3. Estimates of National Costs of the Medical Liability System.[10]

the graph represent billions. This data allows us to draw some interesting conclusions.

Firstly, lawyers' fees nearly equaled indemnity payments to plaintiffs, with $5.72 billion disbursed to patients compared to $4.13 billion for administrative costs. This means that for every $100 awarded to injured patients, $42 went toward lawyers' fees and administrative expenses.

As demonstrated by these figures, victory in a medical malpractice suit comes at a steep price for patients and families. While this might initially appear reasonable, a closer examination reveals a more troubling question: *Who ultimately bears the burden for all these financial awards?*

The immediate answer, of course, is insurance companies. But who ultimately bears the burden of these costs for insurance companies? Once again, the answer is clear: doctors, nurses, medical centers, nursing homes, and others who purchase malpractice coverage.

The correlation between higher payouts and increased insurance premiums is undeniable. In fact, according to the American Medical Association, premiums rose year over year by 29.5% in 2021, slightly down from 31.1% in 2020, which marked the highest increase since 2005.[11] These costs are a significant part of hospitals' and practitioners' overhead.

Faced with escalating expenses, medical providers typically have one of two options: They can either raise service rates or increase the volume of services rendered. For hospitals and nursing homes, this often translates into higher prices. These costs are ultimately borne by patients — either directly through out-of-pocket payments or indirectly via insurance companies through rising premiums, copays, and deductibles. In the case of Medicare, unfortunately, increased costs may lead to higher taxes imposed on the population as a whole to cover these mounting expenses.

Healthcare practitioners, however, face limitations in how much they can increase billing for services. Medicare and the major insurers typically set fixed rates that are non-negotiable. As a result, providers are left with few viable options: They can either accept the reduced payments, increase revenue per patient (often by ordering unnecessary tests and procedures), or see more patients each day to offset the financial shortfall.

And what happens when doctors rush to see more and more patients in order to recapture lost revenue? They may become more prone to errors and carelessness, increasing the likelihood of facing malpractice lawsuits. Thus, malpractice can perpetuate further malpractice!

Over time, it becomes increasingly evident that the primary beneficiaries of this whole fiasco are the lawyers. While injured parties receive just over 50% of settlements, they ultimately bear the brunt of the aftermath: higher taxes, diminished healthcare quality in the future, and higher insurance premiums, copays, and deductibles every year.

This issue takes on a more frightening dimension if we probe further into the data. According to the *Health Affairs* article, the most significant impact of our medical liability system isn't the awards paid to plaintiffs, but rather the extensive use of defensive medicine, which in 2008 alone was estimated to cost nearly $46 billion dollars (in comparison to just under $6 billion in indemnity payments).[10]

Defensive medicine refers to medical practices aimed at reducing the risk of malpractice litigation, often through excessive diagnostic testing. This increased financial burden initially affects private medical insurers, Medicare, and the uninsured. Private medical insurers, of course, pass on these costs through increased premiums, copays, and deductibles while Medicare may need to raise additional funds through taxes and means testing to cover shortfalls.

The result remains the same no matter how you slice the pie: You and I, the American public, are ultimately dipping into our own pocketbooks to fund these lawyers who continue to wreak havoc within our healthcare system. Here's how:

- Doctors work longer hours, practice defensive medicine, and suffer from medical malpractice stress syndrome.
- Patients receive more rushed care and unnecessary tests, resulting in higher costs through increased premiums and taxes.
- Plaintiffs and their families endure years of emotional distress and mourning during legal battles, facing slim odds of success and sharing at least 40% of any settlement with legal professionals.
- Insurers and hospitals transfer their rising costs to the public, often achieving substantial profits despite the financial strain.

Yet somehow, we have allowed these third parties to scapegoat healthcare providers, pointing to poorly conceived and misinterpreted studies of medical errors to divert our focus. Don't misunderstand me — the study of medical errors is crucial, but the data are being cynically manipulated to mislead us.

Once again, doctors and patients find themselves locked in a contentious stance, mere pawns in a game that funnels money out of citizens' pockets and into the coffers of the legal industry. Meanwhile, those actually responsible for delivering care in America are bypassed entirely.

As we sit on opposite sides of the courtroom, grumbling at each other, the wolves are plundering the hen house.

THE BONDS OF ALLYSHIP

Profit-driven decisions are rendering our healthcare system dysfunctional. We've lost sight of what has traditionally bound us together in the doctor-patient relationship. Through the centuries, although the methods of care delivery and the definition of treatment success have evolved significantly, empathy and compassion were steadfast pillars of our relationship — until recently.

Healthcare erodes when trust and faith in this sacred bond deteriorate. In simpler times, it was universally understood that healing requires a mutual exchange, a two-way street in which patients and providers both give of themselves. Today, fears of malpractice and a litigious culture have transformed American healthcare into a self-serving endeavor.

Physicians hoard their knowledge, hesitant to share beliefs or insights for fear that they will be weaponized. We order too many tests, spend too much time on charting to create a defensible story, and are often perceived by those we care for as adversaries lying in wait.

Patients walk into the exam room filled with distrust and worry. They have not only fallen victim to disease and the aging process, but also to a legal system that advises them to be excessively cautious, take notes, and "call immediately if they suspect that they have been wronged."

Throughout this chapter, we have emphasized the financial aspects of the medicolegal system, but we must also consider what cannot be quantified. What happens to ordinary citizens when they lose faith in their doctors? A study published in *PloS One* in 2017 concluded that "From a clinical perspective, patients reported more beneficial health behaviors, less symptoms and higher quality of life and to be more satisfied with treatment when they had higher trust in their health care professional."[12]

Medical malpractice is significantly undermining this trust. However, according to a 2019 *New York Times* article,[13] medical malpractice is contributing little to improve the quality of healthcare. We are giving everything and receiving very little in return.

It's time we put an end to this.

TOWARD BUILDING A BETTER SYSTEM

The goal of this book is not to provide a definitive solution to the medical malpractice crisis. While I lack expertise in crafting legislative or legal policies that could effectively balance the needs of patients and caregivers, the data, as well as the experience of healthcare practitioners and patients, convince me that the current system has been manipulated to serve special interests — primarily lawyers and legal practices. Many potential solutions have been successfully implemented in other countries, which the United States could consider exploring. Let's look at some of their solutions.

Judge versus Jury

One approach is the use of judges rather than juries to adjudicate medical malpractice cases. Several countries, including Germany, the UK, and various Commonwealth nations, have adopted this method. Judges in these systems are highly trained and possess a deep understanding of medicolegal issues. This streamlined approach tends to be more efficient, cost-effective, and rigorous compared to the U.S. system. Experts often argue that judges are better equipped to grasp the nuances and complexities of these cases than untrained juries or nonspecialized professionals.

However, proponents of adopting a judge-centric approach in the United States face a significant hurdle: The Seventh Amendment of the Bill of Rights guarantees the right to a jury trial in civil cases involving amounts greater than $20.

It's All in the Experts

Other countries have focused on the issue of expert witnesses. In the United States, lawyers typically hire and compensate expert witnesses generously, which can potentially influence the objectivity of their testimony due to financial incentives. This practice results in a system where expert witnesses hired by opposing parties present conflicting opinions.

Conversely, in countries like Germany, court-appointed expert witnesses are used. These experts remain impartial as they are compensated regardless of the opinions they express, thereby minimizing any bias toward either party. This system enhances the likelihood that judges receive the most unbiased and objective opinions available. While the United States does employ court-appointed expert witnesses on occasion, it is not yet standard practice.

Planning for Contingencies

Many countries address the issue of excessive litigation by imposing caps on attorneys' fees. One straightforward approach is eliminating the contingency fee system. When attorneys work on contingency, they are taking a chance on the outcome: If successful, they often take a disproportionately large share of the settlement (as high as one third), but if unsuccessful, they receive nothing. While this arrangement reduces financial barriers for victims and families upfront, it also introduces incentives that prioritize financial gain over other considerations.

In contrast, both the UK and Germany routinely prohibit percentage-based contingency fees, leading to lower overall settlement amounts and legal fees. While critics in the United States argue that contingency fees divert significant sums from injured parties and deter lawyers from taking on meritorious cases with lower potential damages, many acknowledge that without this system, the costs of pursuing legal action would be prohibitively high for those seeking justice.

The Loser Pays All

Many people argue that a central problem with the U.S. system is that there is no deterrent to bringing forth frivolous suits. Patients and families are often encouraged to pursue legal action through ubiquitous TV ads and billboards promising minimal financial risk due to contingency fees. Despite the broader societal costs discussed earlier — we all pay the price for the United States' obsession with medical malpractice settlements — the initial risk to potential plaintiffs appears low.

Furthermore, some attorneys and patients exploit the power of nuisance lawsuits, a common occurrence in nursing homes in my experience. In these cases, a patient or lawyer may allege a poor outcome and demand a small settlement from the facility, typically \$10,000 to \$20,000. They know that the high cost of litigation will likely dissuade the nursing home from mounting a defense, leading them to settle regardless of the claim's validity.

In Germany and the UK, however, they operate under a loser-pays system where the unsuccessful party bears the legal fees of the prevailing party. These types of arrangements tend to squash frivolous claims quickly.

While a few states like Alaska and Florida have experimented with similar rules, widespread adoption remains elusive.

To Err Is Human — The No-Fault Approach

Finally, several countries have adopted systems to manage malpractice that resemble those for car accidents or workplace injuries. In these countries, if injuries occurring within the medical system meet specific criteria, they trigger a government payment for a predetermined amount. This approach is common in countries like New Zealand and Sweden.

One major benefit of this system is its efficiency: Payments are streamlined, and patients often receive compensation within months. It also operates at low administrative costs, making it attractive for implementation in countries that adopt it.

I would be remiss in not mentioning that some systems are far more severe about medical malpractice than is the United States. In China, for example medical malpractice is treated as a criminal rather than a civil matter. This means that individuals found guilty not only risk losing their livelihood but also face potential imprisonment. While this contrasts sharply with practices in the United States, a recent case involving ICU nurse Radonda Vaught in 2022, who was convicted of negligent homicide in regard to her treatment of a critically ill patient and sentenced to probation, highlights potential similarities.

We may not be as far from China as we think.

A Price Above Rubies

Ultimately, as a society, we must confront the true cost of maintaining this sprawling medicolegal complex that has engulfed the United States. How much suffering must we endure?

- How many doctors will abandon their practices and close their doors for good?
- How many patients like Francine will perish prematurely in a system that seems to have lost its compassion?
- How many caregivers will endure the strains of Medical Malpractice Stress Syndrome?
- How many community members will discover they can no longer afford insurance or struggle to meet tax and Medicare obligations?

We can only answer such questions if we are willing to follow the money. We must follow the twists and turns that amount to a vast pick-pocketing of the American public and an enrichment of a privileged few.

Lawyers aren't the sole beneficiaries of this broken system. As subsequent chapters will reveal, the creators of electronic medical systems, corporate giants, and even government entities are reaping significant rewards from our broken system.

• • • • • •

Atul Gawande, an American surgeon and writer, stands as one of the most influential figures in contemporary medicine. Through his books and articles, he skillfully weaves his own experiences and also those of his patients.

Amid scrutiny from the American medicolegal system, highlighted by reports like the Institute of Medicine's *To Err is Human*, Dr. Gawande has emerged as a leading advocate for patient safety through thoughtful, scientifically driven, and intelligent system design.

And his storytelling has changed the face of medical practice, notably popularizing the concept of checklists within American culture, as part of and beyond the medical field.

The Checklist Manifesto/Atul Gawande

> *"Even the most expert among us can gain from searching out the patterns of mistakes and failures and putting a few checks in place. But will we do it?"*

In his 2007 article in *The New Yorker*, Atul Gawande recounts a story shared with him by another doctor:

> *"I spoke to Markus Thalmann, the cardiac surgeon on the team that saved the little Austrian girl who had drowned, and learned that a checklist had been crucial to her survival."*

Gawande's 2009 best-selling book, *The Checklist Manifesto*,[14] inspired by this interaction, presents a riveting series of narratives ranging from this high-stakes drowning victim in Australia to Michigan, where a simple cleanliness checklist in intensive care units virtually eradicated a deadly type of hospital infection.

Through these stories, Gawande draws parallels between the impact of checklists in fields like the airline industry, business, and the intricate world of surgical and ICU care. His goal was to introduce the concept of checklists not only to healthcare professionals and safety experts, but also to the broader American public.

In contrast to the finger wagging of the medicolegal complex, Gawande's stories captivated public sentiment and sent shock waves through the patient safety community. He conducted extensive research, including studying the implementation of a 19-item surgical checklist in eight hospitals worldwide. As reported by a *New York Times* article:[15]

> *"The results were startling: The mortality rate fell to 0.8 percent from 1.5 percent, and surgical complications declined to 7 percent from 11 percent. In the decade that ensued, surgical checklists proved effective in diverse settings. In South Carolina, in hospitals that implemented checklists, the 30-day mortality for certain surgical procedures fell to 2.8 percent from 3.4 percent."*

For the last decade, a nonprofit founded by Dr. Gawande has surveyed almost 1,500 hospitals in 94 countries to assess the adoption of surgical checklists.

Atul Gawande is a prime example of how shared storytelling (in this case from doctor) as opposed to adversarial litigation, has profoundly influenced medical error reduction and propelled the patient safety movement.

CHAPTER SEVEN.

Are We Beholden to Our Electronic Mistresses? (Access)

THE ADVENT OF ELECTRONIC MEDICAL RECORDS in the early 2000s promised a revolutionary shift in the delivery of healthcare as we know it. America's hospitals and medical clinics invested billions in high-priced, overly complicated systems that became a windfall for high-tech companies nationwide.

Healthcare providers bore the brunt of this investment, grappling with cumbersome systems that not only disrupted their workflows but also made them the primary drivers of data entry and management. Despite expectations for a streamlined and safer healthcare environment, these promises have largely gone unfulfilled.

Instead, burdened by their electronic taskmasters, they now spend less time with actual patients and more time squinting at computer screens. Not only has this created a further schism in the doctor-patient relationship, it also failed to deliver the anticipated improvements in healthcare quality, cost-efficiency, or safety.

Meanwhile, the massive financial outlay required for these systems has primarily benefited their creators, sellers, and marketers, without yielding substantial benefits within the medical system itself. We have given everything and received nothing.

A BRIEF HISTORY OF ELECTRONIC MEDICAL RECORDS

In 2004, my medical practice underwent a dramatic transformation in the span of a single week, converting from a handwritten medical chart to a fully electronic medical record (EMR) system. During this transition, our corporate employer "generously" allowed clinicians double the usual time to see each patient. This extra time, however, came with a daunting expectation — we were expected to transfer thousands of pages of medical information written in decades of hand-collated charts into a cumbersome and often unintuitive electronic system.

The task was so monumental that many clinicians took years to fully adapt. We faced the overwhelming challenge of quickly distilling vast amounts of medical data during patient exams, frequently needing to make split-second decisions about which less-critical information to omit. Countless unpaid nights and weekends were spent striving to ensure a smooth transition while minimizing disruption to our patients' care.

Despite our efforts, we received no additional compensation for this extensive work, and, in fact, many experienced reduced bonuses due to decreased productivity during the transition. We effectively became unpaid laborers in the push toward implementation.

While our practice was ahead of its time in adopting electronic records as early as 2004, the groundwork for America's electronic medical records had been laid decades earlier. The Mayo Clinic in Rochester Minnesota was one of the first real-time users of EMRs in the 1960s.[1] While the benefits were recognized early on, the high costs of such systems, and necessary hardware, initially limited implementation among most medical practices.

Beginning in the 1970s, the federal government became one of the earliest users of electronic medical records, with Veteran's Administration hospitals leading the way with the implementation of the VistA system.[2] By 1991, the Institute of Medicine recognized electronic medical records as one of its seven key recommendations, and in 2004, the Office of the National Coordinator (ONC) of Health Information Technology was established in Washington.

Legislation further integrated EMRs into the U.S. healthcare system with the Health Information Technology for Economic and Clinical Health (HITECH) Act in 2009. This act provided additional payments to providers who demonstrated "meaningful use" of electronic health records (EHRs). Meaningful use is a program run by the Centers for Medicare & Medicaid Services (CMS) that encourages healthcare providers to use electronic health record technology in ways that benefit patients and providers. HIPAA regulations were also amended to address the electronic protection of health information maintained by EHRs.

Two significant factors fueled the EMR revolution of the 1990s. First, advancements in computer-based technology reduced costs and expanded capabilities, making it feasible for physicians' offices and hospitals to afford the necessary hardware for such systems.[3] Second, systems originally developed and used primarily by governmental institutions or academic centers became commercially accessible to all through for-profit third-party vendors. In fact, by 2014, the top five private vendors controlled more than 50% of the market share.[4]

THE GOVERNMENT STEPS IN

While many agreed that, in theory, electronic medical records were essential for transforming medical care, the HITECH Act placed the direction and control of this transformation squarely in the hands of the government. While the efforts to define "meaningful use" were commendable, the legislation also established a framework of rules, incentives, and penalties that ultimately drove the rise of the multibillion-dollar electronic medical industry that exists today.

First, to assess whether an EMR met the criteria for meaningful use, the government needed to designate certifying bodies. These external entities, known as ONC-Authorized Certification Bodies, added another layer of administrative oversight and fees to our healthcare system. Companies like Drummond Group and Leidos, Inc., have profited significantly from this certification business.

Second, the HITECH Act introduced a range of rewards and penalties to encourage compliance with the electronic transformation. Beginning in 2011, the government offered incentives as high as $18,000 to healthcare practices that achieved meaningful use compliance.[5] While these incentives were crucial for practices willing to adopt this new mandate, starting in 2015, penalties were imposed in the form of reduced Medicare and Medicaid reimbursements for practices that lagged in the implementation of the technology. Over the years, the program has evolved to incorporate newer requirements as outlined in meaningful use stages 2 and 3.

To give due credit, this legislation has significantly increased the use of electronic medical records. Between 2011 to 2018, the U.S. government allocated over $30 billion in incentives to promote meaningful use, resulting in over 95% of eligible hospitals and 60% of office-based physicians achieving this standard by 2016.[6]

The costs of this transformation, however, are not borne solely by the government. The broader healthcare system is footing the bill. Expenditures on EMRs grew at an annual rate of 5.4% between 2015 and 2019, reaching a total of $14.5 billion. Projections indicate spending could rise to $9.9 billion in 2024 alone.[7]

The larger question now is whether this substantial investment is genuinely enhancing American healthcare outcomes. Is this big bet paying off?

WHAT IS THE RETURN ON INVESTMENT?

One could make a compelling argument that investing in a better system to track, record, and manage individuals' healthcare needs is justified. While the need for improvement is obvious, if we are funneling billions into the hands of largely private businesses — such as electronic medical records vendors, certifying agencies, and meaningful use consultants — we must ensure that these investments are genuinely benefiting healthcare outcomes.

So, are they?

Several studies have tackled the question of whether electronic medical records improve care quality and reduce costs, but unfortunately, they offer conflicting conclusions:

- A 2020 study in *JAMA Open* found that in simulations, electronic health records failed to identify one in three potentially harmful drug interactions and other medical errors.[8]
- Research published in *JAMA Network Open* analyzing closed malpractice claims from 2015 to 2021 indicated that EMRs contributed to diagnostic errors in 61% of claims.[9]
- According to a 2015 meta-analysis in *Critical Care Medicine,* electronic interventions did not show a substantial effect on mortality, length of stay, or cost on hospital or ICU stays.[10]
- In 2023, the neurosurgery department at the University of California San Francisco conducted a study to measure the amount of time their residents spent logged into record systems during shifts. The study found that, on average, each resident spent 20 hours per shift logged on to the EHR.[11]
- A 2016 observational study published in *Medicine* using state inpatient data bases showed: "Patients receiving medical and surgical care

at hospitals with no EHR system have similar outcomes compared to patients seeking care at hospitals with a full EHR system, after controlling for important confounders."[12]

- A 2016 *European Journal of Public Health* study showed that EHR use can result in a reduced documentation time, a higher guideline adherence, and a lower number of medication errors.[13]

While numerous studies and meta-analyses present both positive and negative findings, it becomes evident that any potential benefits of EMRs are likely minimal. Moreover, the transition to electronic systems has introduced new types of errors, contributed to physician burnout, and raised concerns about cybersecurity risks and costs. To put it more bluntly, electronic medical records are anything but a slam dunk when it comes to quality or affordability. Despite this, a thriving industry has emerged around these systems, proving to be highly lucrative regardless of their actual impact on healthcare outcomes.

WHY WE HAVEN'T INVESTED WISELY

Let's start by examining the low-hanging fruit. Reliability issues and downtime are major concerns with electronic medical records that often lead to significant financial losses in healthcare. One study found that 96% of organizations experienced at least one unplanned EHR downtime,[14] with another showing that 70% of these downtimes lasted eight hours or more.[15] More alarmingly, some of this downtime is caused by cyberattacks that not only incur financial costs for the organizations but also jeopardize the security of patient data. A 2023 study revealed that U.S. healthcare organizations suffered an average of 1,410 weekly cyberattacks per organization in 2022, marking an 86% increase from the previous year.[16]

Furthermore, we confront a staggering interoperability challenge within our healthcare system. Electronic medical systems fail to allow communication among hospitals, clinicians, and medical facilities. While it's widely acknowledged that improving this interoperability would enhance care, the incentives are misaligned.[17]

Electronic medical records systems are designed by their creators not to facilitate record transfers between different systems, but to encourage organizations to purchase their own proprietary technology. Hospitals are reluctant to share medical records with other institutions, preferring to retain patient traffic within their own facilities. Similarly, doctors' offices are hesitant to allow access to their charts from other offices, aiming to maintain patient loyalty within their practice.

Finally, physicians overwhelmingly dislike electronic medical records and believe they contribute significantly to workplace dissatisfaction. A Stanford poll revealed that 71% of clinicians feel that EMRs strongly contribute to burnout and 59% believe these systems require a complete overhaul.[18] This sentiment is reflected in predictions that by 2025, 75% of healthcare workers plan to leave the profession.[19] Instead of simplifying their work, physicians are voting with their feet and leaving their jobs in frustration. The costs associated with replacing this workforce and mitigating burnout have not been factored into the return-on-investment calculations for EMRs.

Given these complexities and the underlying costs associated with electronic medical records, one might expect a consensus on their overall benefits. Unfortunately, the data remain inconclusive and the debate continues.

THE BIG BUSINESS OF ELECTRONIC HEALTH RECORDS

According to market research company Business Intelligence, the electronic health record market is projected to reach $38.3 billion in 2025,[20] with the lion's share dominated by a handful of large vendors. The KLAS U.S. Hospital EMR Market Share 2019 report highlights Epic EHR and Cerner as leaders in hospital EHR systems, while Epic and Allscripts dominate in ambulatory clinics.[21]

Epic, for example, was founded in 1979 and has experienced rapid growth in recent years. By 2023, Epic employed an estimated 10,000 people and was valued at $7.4 billion, up from $3.5 billion in 2018.[22]

As of the mid-2020s, Epic serves over 600 healthcare organizations and more than 2,800 hospitals worldwide, supporting the care of roughly 300 million patients in the United States — representing the majority of the population.[23] Founder and owner Judith Faulkner's net worth is estimated to be $7.8 billion.[24]

Despite Epic's remarkable growth and the substantial net worth it has generated for its owner, questions persist about the overall benefits to our medical system from such wealth creation. According to most studies, these financial gains have had negligible positive impacts. Billions of dollars have been extracted from government and medical systems to fund these services, with the resulting costs passed down to the American public through taxes, higher prices, copays, and deductibles.

Moreover, these costs are ongoing. A 2022 study revealed that the average medical practice needs to allocate $1,200 per user per year for EHR software updates and changes.[25] This user base isn't solely comprised of the nation's 1.1 million doctors; it also includes support staff, estimated to be between three to five individuals per full-time practicing physician.[26] These figures illustrate how companies like Epic can continue to accrue annual revenues in the range of at least $5 billion.

TOWARD BUILDING A BETTER SYSTEM

While the evidence supporting the benefits of electronic medical records lags, I suspect that much of the reason is our investment in disparate, non-communicative, commercial, and excessively complex systems. These systems are built with profits in mind — either by extracting substantial fees from medical providers or by promising providers the ability to maximize reimbursements from payers. As is often the case in healthcare and beyond, following the money reveals severe misalignments in incentives.

There are several avenues through which we can realign incentives to improve medical care delivery and reduce technology costs. Here are a few suggestions:

VistA for All

Originally known as the Decentralized Hospital Computer Program (DHCP), the roots of VistA (Veterans Health Information Systems and Technology Architecture) likely trace back to the 1960s.[27] This expansive initiative by the Veterans Administration aimed to establish an electronic health record system for the nation's extensive network of veterans' hospitals, emphasizing simplicity, accessibility, and connectivity across facilities nationwide.

Devoid of the bells and whistles of commercial products used for complicated billing issues and meaningful use, this stalwart system has faithfully supported medical students, residents, attending physicians, and VA patients for decades. I vividly recall, as a student, signing onto the system for the first time and becoming proficient within hours.

The system is remarkably user-friendly and practical — it just works.

Efforts to replace the VistA system with updated commercial products in recent years have proven disastrous. According to Edward Meagher, former deputy assistant secretary and deputy CIO at the Department of Veterans Affairs, five years of implementing pilot programs with commercial products resulted in catastrophic outcomes,[28] including the deaths of at least four veterans,[29] harm to hundreds more, a 50% reduction in productivity at the five VA medical centers involved, and wasteful spending nearing $10 billion.

Ultimately, the VA reversed course on these live experiments after realizing the new EMRs failed to meet expectations, opting to revert to the reliable VistA system. I believe it's time for the nation to follow suit. We should discontinue the use of these costly commercial systems and instead adopt an affordable and straightforward solution like VistA. Such a system, government-provided, could incorporate built-in functionality for reporting. It could seamlessly extract information required for government programs like meaningful use with minimal effort, if not automatically.

Interoperability

The interoperability challenge severely hampers the utility of electronic medical records. Interoperability is the ability of health data systems to share and use data securely, regardless of location, to improve patient care and community health. For progress to be made, systems across neighboring, opposing, and even national databases must be able to communicate seamlessly with each other. Full stop. Without interoperability, a significant portion of the potential benefits of EMRs is lost.

The crux of the interoperability issue lies in both technological and cultural barriers. Hundreds of certified electronic medical record products are available, each with its own technology, workflow, and functional capabilities.[30] For these systems to interact effectively, they must be capable of exchanging information using standardized and structured data formats. Regrettably, there currently is no universal standard adopted across the various commercial systems.

Even if a universal standard were established, a significant cultural divide still looms, as noted by Miriam Reisman in 2017:[30]

> *"Perhaps the biggest obstacle facing EHR interoperability is not technological but cultural. As in other industries, interoperability in health care requires the close coordination and collaboration of various stakeholders, including patients, providers, software vendors, legislators, and health information technology (IT) professionals. Yet the U.S. health care delivery system continues to have a culture defined by silos, fragmented processes, and disparate stakeholders, and where data have become more of a commodity and competitive advantage than a basis for coordinated care."*

Simply put, there are compelling reasons why many healthcare entities hesitate to share data with each other. While a clinician's ethical responsibility is to provide the best patient care possible, medical systems prioritize their fiduciary responsibility to shareholders, employees, and boards of directors. Encouraging patients to seek services elsewhere in competing systems runs counter to their financial interests.

Likewise, electronic medical record companies have little incentive to facilitate data sharing across platforms. A 2017 study in *Millbank Quarterly* addresses the issue of information blocking, which is intentionally interfering with the flow of information between different EHR systems. A survey of electronic health information exchange leaders found that half of respondents reported EHR vendors engage in routine information blocking, with an additional 33% acknowledging occasional obstruction.[31] While these figures were somewhat lower for hospitals and healthcare systems (25% routine and 34% occasional), significant barriers persist.

To move forward, mandatory information sharing among all systems is essential. Commercial systems that hinder interoperability should be phased out in favor of a standardized nationwide EMR solution, akin to VistA as discussed earlier, which could effectively address these challenges.

Meaningful Use

This much ballyhooed program has had a slew of unintended consequences. As former American Medical Association (AMA) President Andrew Gurman, MD, succinctly stated, "Prescriptive design, use, and certification demands by the federal government have driven the design of EHRs to focus on CMS reporting requirements, largely ignoring the needs of physicians and patients."[30]

As discussed earlier, this approach has exacerbated physician burnout and contributed to the great resignation of healthcare practitioners. Physicians now spend more time than ever tethered to computer systems and less time providing hands-on patient care. For every hour of clinical work, physicians devote at least two hours to EHR-related tasks.[32]

Regrettably, as is often the case, what gets measured ends up receiving the most attention. While we excel in meeting many of these artificially created quality indicators, the fundamental question remains: Are we truly improving patient outcomes? The data suggest otherwise.

To the government's credit, CMS renamed the EHR Incentive Programs from "meaningful use" to the Medicare and Medicaid Promoting Interoperability Programs in April 2018. This change aimed to transition from the existing requirements of meaningful use to a new phase of EHR measurement, emphasizing interoperability and enhancing patient access to health information.[33] While this shift represents a positive step forward, these programs often place too much burden on physicians while absolving EMR credentialing agencies and vendors of their share of responsibility.

Ultimately, electronic medical records should be designed to better align with the needs of end-users. Rather than simply measuring meaningful use, the focus should be on assessing meaningful usability. The responsibility must shift away from clinicians to foster a more effective and beneficial healthcare system.

Almost Everyone Loses

I opened this chapter by asking if we are indeed beholden to an electronic taskmaster. The answer could not be clearer. The practice of medicine has been transformed through government-backed incentives that funneled money into private ventures and technology. While the initial promise was improved quality, reduced costs, and enhanced efficiency, the outcomes have often been quite the opposite.

- EMRs have not been definitively shown to improve the quality of care.

- EMRs have not conclusively demonstrated cost savings.
- EMRs have placed a significant time and administrative burden on physicians, exacerbating burnout.
- EMRs have already cost our medical system billions and will continue to incur hefty annual expenses.
- When large entities like the VA tried to transition from a simplified EMR to a commercial one, they were forced to abandon the effort after five years due to adverse outcomes.

The sole beneficiaries in this scenario are the companies that developed and now sell the technology to operate these systems. Neither doctors, nor patients, nor our healthcare system at large have emerged as winners. We have paid dearly and gained little in return.

......

Almost every doctor I know has, at some point, delved into the pages of Samuel Shem's book *The House of God*. For those of us who read it during training, it was a badge of honor to find solace in someone who understands and reflects our shared experiences.

This novel offers a deeply cynical portrayal of medical training, following protagonist Dr. Roy Basch as he navigates the tumultuous and often PTSD-inducing journey familiar to many who have traversed the path of medical training. For me, the book drew laughter and tears, sometimes at the same time.

Set in the 1970s, the highly technological and administratively burdened world of today's healthcare system would have been beyond the imagination of the fictional characters originally created by Dr. Shem (the pen name for psychiatrist Stephen Bergman). This stark contrast is evident in his subsequent novel, *Man's 4th Best Hospital*,[34] where Dr. Basch, Fat Man, and their cohorts confront a world that has dramatically evolved since their earlier adventures.

Man's 4th Best Hospital/Dr. Samuel Shem (Stephen Bergman)

Years after the fictional trials of Dr. Roy Basch in *The House of God*, he returns to work at a clinic affiliated with what is cynically dubbed as

Man's 4th Best Hospital, dedicated to the future of medicine.[34] Unlike the challenges he faced in the tumultuous 1970s and 1980s, a new threat to the human element of medicine has emerged. Instead of battling the depersonalization and relentless demands of his residency decades ago, he now confronts a new and insidious adversary in the field: technology.

What unfolds is both a heartbreaking as well as an amusing explanation of how the medical profession, through the eyes of a seasoned physician, has transformed over the past three decades. Set in contemporary academic medicine, this fictional novel portrays the struggle against the encroachment of technology and corporate greed perpetuated by a new generation of corporate overlords.

Like *The House of God*, this novel exemplifies what author Samuel Shem describes as "Fiction as Resistance." In Shem's own words:

> *"So doctors somehow have to find a way — and under pressure, we might — to stick together. Doctors have to make an alliance with nurses, and other health care workers, and patients. That's a solid group of people representing themselves in terms of what we think is good health care. The profession we love has been taken over, with us sitting there in front of screens all day, doing data entry in a computer factory."*

Shem's fictional works exemplify the healing essence of narrative. They illustrate how narratives can be used not just to depict reality, but also to convey and exchange knowledge, to resist through storytelling, and to forge alliances. He explains how we can become allies.

The House of God played a pivotal role in shaping a generation of physicians characterized by empathy, humility, and humanity. *Man's 4th Best Hospital* serves as a reminder amidst the overwhelming pressures of modern medicine and technology, ensuring that these essential qualities are not lost. Shem's stories have profoundly influenced both the medical profession and the broader world.

CHAPTER EIGHT.

Have We Been Legislated Out? (Incentives)

THE GOVERNMENT IS NOT HERE TO SAVE US; rather, its legislative actions have increasingly distanced doctors from their patients. Accountable care organizations exemplify this trend, where physicians are compelled to act as gatekeepers, often perceived as controlling access to care and bearing the brunt of community dissatisfaction when issues arise.

Furthermore, burdensome legislation that increases compliance and the adoption of meaningful use of electronic medical records has accelerated the decline of private practices. This has driven consolidation into larger healthcare systems, a shift from nonprofit to for-profit medicine, and a buying spree by private equity and venture capital.

In this chapter, we delve deeper into specific policies that illustrate a troubling trajectory from well-intentioned legislation to the exclusion of doctors, the essential stakeholders in healthcare delivery. How does governmental policy obstruct medical practice and widen the gap between doctors and patients? Are these policies inadvertently legislating doctors and patients out of the healthcare system?

And crucially, what remedies can be pursued to address these challenges?

THE FALSE CLAIMS ACT

Fraud in our healthcare system is indisputable, involving not only administrators and healthcare systems but also occasionally doctors and other medical professionals. While every profession has its bad actors, this reality has spurred sweeping legislation aimed at combating fraud but often yielding unintended consequences.

The False Claims Act (FCA) originally enacted in 1863 to address fraud among defense contractors during the Civil War,[1] imposes severe penalties on individuals who knowingly submit false claims to the U.S. government. Violators may be liable for triple damages plus penalties adjusted for inflation. Additionally, whistleblowers — private individuals — can initiate claims on behalf of the government against those suspected of fraudulent activity.

Settlements and judgments under the False Claims Act exceeded $2.2 billion in the fiscal year ending Sept. 30, 2022.[2] While the act serves to protect public funds, its broad application and punitive measures can inadvertently harm legitimate healthcare providers and exacerbate challenges in the healthcare industry.

While the FCA has been broadly applied outside the realm of healthcare, physician liability extends beyond the traditional definition of "knowingly." Physicians or healthcare entities can meet the "knowing" requirement by demonstrating "reckless disregard" or "deliberate ignorance" of the facts or circumstances surrounding a violation. Shockingly, the FCA has even penalized physicians who inadvertently received overpayments from Medicare and Medicaid, citing failure to promptly repay the government fast enough.

Why does this cause problems? The sheer volume of rules and regulations makes compliance exceedingly difficult for doctors. Coding accurately becomes a formidable task, and audits frequently reveal instances of upcoding, a type of healthcare fraud that occurs when a provider submits inaccurate billing codes to an insurance company for a medical procedure or treatment to increase reimbursement. This is universally true regardless of who is audited. While mastering human anatomy is daunting enough, navigating thousands of diagnostic codes, comprehending intricate evaluation and management scoring, and correctly applying modifiers can border on the impossible.

In 2020, Medicare estimated a coding error rate of approximately 6.8% for Medicare Part C services rendered between July 1, 2019, and June 30, 2020, as illustrated in Table 4.[3] In 2022, the coding error rate was approximately 7.5% for services rendered between July 1, 2020 and June 30, 2021.

In such a complex system, a 7.5% error rate might seem acceptable initially. However, when considering the potential ramifications — such as triple damages under the False Claims Act and additional inflation-adjusted fines — the risks associated with human error can be catastrophic for medical practices. Aware of this risk, clinicians often opt to

Program	2019 Improper Payment Rate	2019 Improper Payments	2020 Improper Payment Rate	2020 Improper Payments
Medicare FFS	7.25%	$28.91	6.27%	$25.74
Medicare Part C	7.87%	$16.73	6.78%	$16.27
Medicare Part D	0.76%	$0.61	1.15%	$0.93
Medicaid	14.90%*	$57.36*	21.36%*	$86.49*
CHIP	15.83%*	$2.74*	27.00%*	$4.78*

*Medicaid and CHIP 2020 estimated improper payments are not comparable to years prior to 2019, due to the reintegration of the PERM eligibility

TABLE 4. FY 2020 Estimated Improper Payment Rates and Improper Payments.[3]

downcode to mitigate potential liabilities, billing at a lower level than what was provided.

Yet downcoding brings its own set of challenges. Practices, already burdened with compliance costs and competing against privately owned medical centers, rely on accurate coding to secure necessary funds. Moreover, intentionally downcoding to evade Medicare scrutiny violates federal regulations like the anti-kickback statute and could be construed as inducement.[4]

In other words, you are damned if you do and damned if you don't.

THE ANTI-KICKBACK STATUTE

The anti-kickback statute (AKS) is a criminal law that strictly prohibits the knowing exchange of remuneration intended to incentivize patient referrals or the generation of business related to services payable by federal healthcare programs.[5] Violations of this statute can lead to severe civil and criminal penalties, including fines, imprisonment, exclusion from federal healthcare programs, and financial penalties of up to $50,000 per kickback, plus three times the remuneration amount. Claims submitted to Medicare or Medicaid in violation of the anti-kickback statute are treated under the False Claims Act, regardless of the defendant's intent.[6]

The necessity of such laws is unequivocal. As a primary care physician practicing in the community, I often encountered situations in which there was a fine line between legitimate practices, such as a nursing home hiring a medical director to enhance quality of care, and improper activities, such as offering excessive stipends solely to encourage that same physician to refer patients. This unethical practice, which I witnessed frequently, underscores the critical need to eliminate such perverse incentives from healthcare operations.

However, the unintended consequences of such laws without appropriate nuance creates situations detrimental to doctors, patients, and society as a whole. A prime example is the impact on physician-owned hospitals. Under the ethos of the anti-kickback statute, the Affordable Care Act imposed stringent restrictions on physician-owned hospitals[7,8] that were nearly impossible to comply with, resulting in the acquisition or change of ownership of nearly a quarter of these institutions.[9] The rationale behind these prohibitions was to prevent physician self-referral practices and the potential for increased financial incentives through kickbacks.

Contrary to these concerns, studies have demonstrated several advantages associated with physician-owned hospitals:

- Commercial negotiated prices and cash prices in physician-owned hospitals were approximately one-third lower than their competitors for eight common services.[10]
- Physician-owned hospitals foster greater physician engagement, deliver higher-quality care, and achieve better patient satisfaction scores, lower costs, and improve infection rates compared to non-physician-owned competitors.[11]
- Interestingly, large hospital systems that are not owned by physicians are not subject to similar self-referral restrictions and can even mandate that contracted physicians refer patients exclusively to their facilities.[12]

These findings challenge the blanket application of restrictive laws without considering nuanced outcomes and suggest that some regulations may inadvertently hinder beneficial healthcare practices.

Finally, the government acknowledges that anti-kickback laws can sometimes create unsustainable scenarios that result in unnecessary costs to our healthcare system. In response, certain safe harbor rules have been established for specific industries and situations. However, these safe harbor provisions that define payment practices that are not considered offenses under the law often become targets for manipulation by third parties seeking to exploit loopholes in the system. As succinctly stated by Madelaine Feldman in *MDedge Rheumatology* in 2023:[13]

> *"During the 1990s, a number of safe harbor provisions under the AKS were instituted for certain payments to health insurance companies, PBMs (Pharmacy Benefits Managers), and other providers. The thinking was that these payments needed a safe harbor because, although they might meet the statutory definition of "kickbacks," they were beneficial because they would reduce the cost of care and, more specifically, the prices of drugs.*
>
> *"While well-intentioned, those safe harbors now protect a system of such perverse incentives that patients are whipsawed back and forth onto drugs that are the most profitable for the PBMs, who create the annual list of insurance covered drugs (i.e., the formulary). It is clear now that protected kickbacks, in the form of rebates and fees paid by pharmaceutical manufacturers to PBMs, determine what drugs will be on the formulary. PBMs then use utilization management tools such as step therapy to force patients to take those drugs first. Consequently, safe harbor protection from the AKS allows manufacturers to buy market share at the expense of patient's health."*

As a result, money intended for healthcare providers ends up diverted to third-party business entities. A process that enriches pharmacy benefit managers while doctors and patients bear the losses. Again!

STARK LAWS

As defined by the Office of the Inspector General, the Physician Self-Referral Law, also known as the Stark law, prohibits physicians from referring patients to receive Medicare or Medicaid payable "designated health services" from entities where the physician or an immediate family member has a financial interest, unless an exception applies.[5] These designated health services include:

- Clinical laboratory services.

- Physical therapy, occupational therapy, and outpatient speech-language pathology services.
- Radiology and certain other imaging services.
- Radiation therapy services and supplies.
- DME and supplies.
- Parenteral and enteral nutrients, equipment, and supplies.
- Prosthetics, orthotics, and prosthetic devices and supplies.
- Home health services.
- Outpatient prescription drugs.
- Inpatient and outpatient hospital services.

Government regulations like the Stark law are designed with clear intentions, aiming to prevent clinicians from self-referring patients for potentially lucrative services without oversight. However, despite these intentions, the law has had unintended and damaging consequences.

Unfortunately, what qualifies as a self-referral can be complicated, and like the anti-kickback law, intent is not taken into consideration. Consequently, many practices and physicians may unknowingly violate the Stark law. Common scenarios include:[14]

- Poorly structured deals involving healthcare businesses providing designated health services.
- Alternative payment models that link physician payments to volume or value of payment referrals (e.g., pay-for-performance, gainsharing).
- Untracked compensation arrangements, whether monetary or non-monetary.
- Technical violations or noncompliance issues, including documentation deficiencies.
- Oversight issues like failing to sign or renew a contact appropriately.
- Accidental omissions of elements required by legal exceptions in agreements.
- Failure to conduct business in strict accordance with written agreements.

Violating these laws can lead to severe penalties under the False Claims Act, including substantial fines and repayment of up to three times the amount of government overpayments.

Both the Stark and anti-kickback laws pose challenges for physicians and medical systems seeking to adopt new payment models that encourage closer coordination among healthcare providers, due to concerns about potential penalties.[15]

OVERREACHING STATE LAWS THAT DICTATE PRACTICE

Furthermore, if federal restrictions were not complicated enough, state governments have increasingly intruded in the exam room, imposing restrictions on what physicians can discuss with patients regarding certain topics. This interference becomes particularly contentious when addressing two specific issues: firearms and women's reproductive rights.

Florida notably led the way in 2011 by enacting what are often referred to as physician gag laws. Under the Firearm Owners' Privacy Act, physicians were prohibited from asking patients about guns in their homes unless there was a direct threat to the patient's medical care or public safety.[16] Although this law was overturned by the courts in 2017, similar legislation was introduced in five states (Indiana, North Carolina, North Dakota, Ohio, and Texas) in 2015,[16] none of which have been enacted to date. It's important to highlight that the National Rifle Association (NRA), yet another third-party with a significant stake in the outcome, has strongly advocated these laws.

Women's reproductive rights have been significantly affected by the issue of gag laws, particularly concerning birth control and abortion. In 2019, the Department of Health and Human Services issued a Final Rule that "impose[d] a gag on the medical profession that would have practitioners in the Title X program direct pregnant women toward continuing a pregnancy to term — regardless of what a patient actually wants (the 'Gag Requirement')."[17]

Many of these gag laws not only regulate discussions within the exam room but also compel physicians to provide information or advice that may contradict their own beliefs or lack empirical support. For example, a law in South Carolina mandated physicians discuss a purported link between abortion and suicide, despite insufficient data supporting such a connection. Although in *Planned Parenthood Minn. ND, SD v Rounds* this case ultimately was overturned, the intent to restrict physician speech is obvious.

Such governmental mandates undermine the trust essential in the doctor-patient relationship. How can patients rely on physicians who must prioritize governmental directives, often influenced by third parties with overarching economic and political agendas, over their professional judgment and ethical obligations?

I WAS LEGISLATED OUT

My personal experience of not only dealing with the medicolegal system but also with being legislated out of practice is not uncommon. It began with the implementation of meaningful use requirements. My practice invested tens of thousands of dollars to adopt these systems to avoid Medicare and Medicaid penalties. However, these systems, inherently cumbersome and often designed without consideration for a physician's workflow, completely altered the dynamics of patient care in my exam room.

Instead of focusing on direct patient interaction — making eye contact, observing cues — we found ourselves glued to computer screens, navigating through irrelevant background data, and constantly addressing pop-up alerts and alarms. The traditional culture of the exam room, honed over centuries by seasoned clinicians, was disrupted. Already pressed for time, we now faced even greater pressures. Frustration mounted as we struggled with electronic systems to perform routine tasks we once managed seamlessly.

HIPAA regulations, intended to safeguard privacy and rights, instead became another barrier between our offices and their patients and families. Suddenly, longstanding relationships required us to alter how we communicated with family members, often leading to denials of information requests due to inadequate documentation.

Meanwhile, Medicare audits became a constant challenge. The introduction of prepayment "target and educate" audits intensified scrutiny on physicians, creating a sense of being under a microscope where one misstep could lead to severe consequences. Through numerous audits, I discovered Medicare's preference for coding visits at the lowest possible levels. Despite meticulous coding and external audits, disagreements often arose between Medicare and our professional coders hired to ensure accuracy.

Navigating these complexities became even more perilous when advised by coders to downgrade submitted claims. Failing to promptly notify Medicare in such cases risked severe and punitive penalties under the False Claims Act.

These laws and regulations made it clear to me as a physician that not only was I under intense scrutiny, but also that the government was eager to impose penalties regardless of the presence of malicious intent. The anti-kickback and Stark laws underscored that even unintentional missteps could lead to severe consequences.

For many physicians, the only viable response has been to consider leaving the field of medicine altogether or to opt out of Medicare and Medicaid regulations. Although the complexities of the latter decision are extensive and require legal guidance and compliance expertise, many have chosen this path. Personally, I took this route when I transitioned from a group private practice to starting my own concierge practice in which I no longer accepted Medicare payments and thus avoided stifling regulations. While some may perceive this move as driven by financial motives, many physicians have pursued this route to escape the burdens of government compliance and avoid being acquired by private equity.

Ultimately, physicians are making decisions they feel they must make to navigate a challenging regulatory landscape and preserve their professional autonomy.

TOWARD BUILDING A BETTER SYSTEM

As mentioned earlier, it's understandable that the government aims to safeguard public funds from misuse. However, the current legal landscape has inadvertently made it increasingly challenging to provide cost-effective, efficient, and patient-centered care. To address this issue, we need to develop a system that not only acknowledges but also respects the nuances involved in healthcare delivery.

Punishment Must Match Intent

While it's evident that the punitive measures of the False Claims Act and anti-kickback laws serve as a deterrent, they also pose a significant barrier to well-intentioned physicians who are striving to innovate within the healthcare system. Amid the myriad federal and state compliance requirements, the potential for unintentional violations — whether through self-referral of designated health services or coding errors leading to inflated Medicare bills — is alarmingly high.

When penalties amount to three times the reimbursement, it sends a stark message to practitioners: Comply strictly or face severe consequences. Unfortunately, the criteria for what constitutes "knowingly" submitting a false claim remains ambiguously defined. Instead of scrutinizing every detail of complex regulations when errors occur, we should place greater emphasis on intent. Accidental mistakes should prompt straightforward repayment and require proper training to prevent recurrence.

By focusing on intent and providing clearer guidelines, we can foster an environment that supports innovation while ensuring compliance with necessary regulations in healthcare.

Simplify, Simplify, Simplify

Many large hospital systems and physician practices employ extensive teams of billers and coders who spend countless hours each week meticulously reviewing medical charts. Physicians themselves require ongoing training in billing and coding practices, often needing regular refresher courses. Electronic medical record companies continuously develop more sophisticated — and costly — products aimed at maximizing revenue capture.

The current system is unnecessarily complex. Simplifying billing and coding by significantly reducing the number of codes and billing levels could streamline operations. Perhaps a straightforward reimbursement scale based on simple, intermediate, or complex care levels, each defined by clear and standardized criteria, could be implemented.

Every dollar spent on billing and coding represents wasted resources. Simplifying these processes could potentially reduce administrative burdens and allow healthcare providers to focus more on patient care rather than navigating convoluted reimbursement systems.

The Benefits of Self-Referral

As we've discussed earlier, physician-run hospitals and clinics often demonstrate better cost-effectiveness and outcomes. However, for these entities to thrive, restrictions on self-referral need to be eased. Surgeons should have the flexibility to refer surgical patients to hospitals or surgical centers in which they have ownership stakes. The stringent regulations imposed on physician-owned hospitals by the Affordable Care Act should be reconsidered.

Moreover, to align with the government's vision of healthcare reform, accountable care organizations and other quality-improvement structures should be exempt from laws like Stark and others that restrict internal referrals. This flexibility is crucial for enhancing overall quality and reducing healthcare costs.

In a positive step forward, in November 2020, the Centers for Medicare & Medicaid Services finalized exceptions to the Stark law to support value-based care models. Concurrently, the Office of Inspector General established safe harbors under the anti-kickback statute aimed at fostering the growth of value-based care initiatives across healthcare providers.[18]

......

Numerous solutions have been proposed to address our healthcare challenges, but true revolutionary change must challenge entrenched third-party interests. Government interventions, as illustrated in this discussion, often lead to unintended consequences that drive a wedge between doctors and patients, prompt physicians to leave the field, and contribute to the increasing influence of private equity in medicine.

In my view, the solution lies outside the current political system. Real change will only happen when the primary stakeholders — doctors and patients — unite and demand a system that serves their interests. Building a stronger alliance between doctors and patients is essential; we need to feel united in our goals.

It's worth acknowledging that some of the world's most stable and cost-effective healthcare systems are universal government-run models. Countries like Canada and the United Kingdom have faced challenges but have effectively managed costs and minimized profit-driven healthcare practices prevalent in the United States.

England's National Health Service (NHS) is frequently referenced as a potential model for healthcare reform in America. Interestingly, the NHS, the UK's version of universal healthcare, faced significant opposition when it was first proposed. Dr. A.J. Cronin's fictional tale, *The Citadel,* sparked a revolution that brought together key stakeholders and demonstrated the power of literature in healthcare reform — ultimately leading to the establishment of the NHS.

The Citadel/Dr. A.J. Cronin

A.J. Cronin, a Scottish-born physician who rose to prominence as a novelist in the 1920s, achieved widespread acclaim with his most famous work, *The Citadel*, published in 1937.[19] Set in Wales and London during the 1920s and 1930s, the novel follows the journey of an idealistic young doctor grappling with a corrupt and inefficient healthcare system. *The Citadel* not only critiqued the state of medicine at the time, but also foreshadowed significant trends in modern medicine, such as evidence-based practice and continuous medical education.

While there is debate over whether Cronin intended the novel as a social commentary on healthcare, it undoubtedly played a role in catalyzing public sentiment. The book's popularity contributed to the momentum that led to the establishment of Britain's National Health Service (NHS) in 1948. Through its exploration of social and health inequalities, *The Citadel* resonated deeply with a broad cross-section of English society.

The roots of the NHS can be traced back to earlier calls for reform, such as those by socialist Beatrice Webb in 1909 and the establishment of the Socialist Medical Association in 1930. It was not until 1946, following World War II, that Health Minister Aneurin Bevan presented the NHS Bill to Parliament. Notably, both Cronin and Bevan had connections to Tredegar Cottage Hospital in Wales, which served as a foundational model for the NHS. Their paths likely crossed.[20]

Despite facing criticism from fellow doctors and politicians, Cronin's literary influence sparked a revolutionary movement in both the practice and funding of medical care in the UK. His writings inspired a profound call for change that reshaped healthcare delivery and accessibility in Britain.

PART THREE.

Toward Building a Better System

IT ALL STARTED ON A GOLF COURSE IN DENVER the afternoon of Friday, Sept. 23, 1955.[1] President Dwight D. Eisenhower initially dismissed his chest pain as indigestion from his lunch — a hamburger with Bermuda onions. However, after awakening with severe chest pain shortly after midnight, he was diagnosed the next day with a heart attack.

Dr. Paul Dudley White, a renowned cardiologist and co-founder of the American Heart Association in 1924, was among Eisenhower's physicians. Rather than simply treating Eisenhower's symptoms, Dr. White recognized the importance of addressing lifestyle factors to prevent future heart problems. He collaborated closely with Eisenhower to implement a comprehensive cardiac rehabilitation program including dietary changes, exercise, and stress-management techniques.

Together, Dr. White and Eisenhower raised awareness about heart disease and promoted healthy living practices. Eisenhower, leveraging his public platform, advocated preventive measures such as regular exercise and balanced diet. This partnership between doctor and patient had a profound impact on public health awareness and cardiovascular medicine.

When doctors and patients work together, amazing things can happen.

So far in this book, I've dedicated significant effort to highlighting the flaws in our healthcare system and how third parties have exploited them for maximum profit. Our attempts to overhaul the medical system have been notably unsuccessful. According to the Peterson-KFF Health

System Tracker, healthcare spending was $74.1 billion in 1970. By 2000, expenditures had soared to around $1.4 trillion, and by 2021, they had tripled to $4.3 trillion.[2] Despite this massive investment, a 2019 brief from the Commonwealth Fund revealed that the United States consistently achieves poorer health outcomes and spends more on healthcare compared to other high-income nations, largely due to extensive use of medical technology and higher prices.[3]

Physicians and patients, as primary stakeholders, have struggled to drive meaningful change in this broken system. In a 2009 article on *The Health Care Blog*, Rahul Parikh questioned the relevance of the American Medical Association (the largest physician lobbying organization in the United States), noting that its membership had dwindled to less than a third of all physicians nationally:[4]

> *"Only time will tell, but given it sinking numbers and traditional resistance to change and innovation in the delivery of health care in the wake of a groundswell of support for change, it's hard not to see this grand old institution of American medicine slowing getting sick and slipping into critical condition."*

Even though posed nearly 17 years ago, his question remains relevant today. Many physicians still feel powerless to effectively advocate for change in our clearly dysfunctional healthcare system. While physicians recognize that our patients are not receiving adequate care, consensus on the necessary next steps often proves elusive.

Similarly, patient advocacy groups have struggled to counteract the overwhelming impact of healthcare inflation and declining quality. Despite advances in medical transparency, the e-patient movement, and peer-to-peer health initiatives, there remains a palpable sense that we have yet to make significant progress against entrenched interests.

To move forward and bring about revolutionary change, these key stakeholders must unite and learn to speak in a singular powerful voice. However, this necessitates viewing each other as allies rather than adversaries. Part Three of this book will discuss how reducing the intimacy gap and shared storytelling can catalyze genuine political and structural reforms.

CHAPTER NINE.

The Intimacy Gap

IF YOU SEARCH "DOCTOR-PATIENT INTIMACY" on Google, you'll find numerous articles discussing and rightly prohibiting sexual relationships between physicians and those under their care. No other form of intimacy is discussed. The reason is straightforward: We have no concept of what mutual non-physical intimacy should entail in this context. The consequences of the lack of consideration are significant.

Patients are expected to divulge their deepest secrets in the exam room, exposing not just their souls but also their bodies. This exchange, crucial for diagnosis and treatment, feels appropriate in the moment of clinical necessity and decision-making, but it is one-sided.

However, on a global scale, to repair the damage inflicted by the destructive forces outlined in Part One that are eroding the doctor-patient relationship, healthcare providers must learn to bridge this intimacy gap; it can no longer be unilateral. Only then can we become allies in the fight to reclaim our medical system. True grassroots change in healthcare will only come to fruition when we, the primary stakeholders, unite and wield our collective power.

The first time I witnessed such profound intimacy between a doctor and patient, my training had conditioned me to view such raw displays of emotion as vulnerability. It took years of practice for me to not only forgive that doctor, but to embrace the humility required to be intimate.

THE HAND HOLDER

When the residents labeled Dr. Foster a "hand holder," it was far from a term of endearment; rather, it conveyed how much we dreaded caring for his patients. It wasn't just his indecisive approach to decision-making, but also his excessively sentimental bedside manner. Despite his popularity among patients, many of us felt the urge to leave the room whenever he spoke.

I vividly recall my final encounter with Dr. Foster. I was a third-year resident, accompanying him on rounds in the ICU. We assessed a gentleman on life support with failing kidneys and heart. After completing his notes, Dr. Foster and I approached the waiting wife, her eyes filled with tears as she shared that the family had decided to withdraw life support. Dr. Foster tightly held her hand, gazing deeply into her eyes. He begged her: "Don't give up yet. I feel like I could have done so much more!"

Moved, the wife gently touched Dr. Foster's cheek before embracing him.

"Doctor. Don't blame yourself. You did all you could. It's time for him to go."

I felt a pang of discomfort. How had Dr. Foster become the focal point of this interaction instead of taking on a more appropriate role of comforting the grieving wife? I couldn't help feeling that I never wanted to work with Dr. Foster again — a wish that, although it came true, did not block his memory from resurfacing unexpectedly years later.

Walter and Sarah were among my most cherished patients. Despite their frail bodies, worn by 70 years of life's challenges, their spirits remained remarkably vibrant. They greeted me in the office with warmth and respect, uplifting the entire medical team.

A year earlier, Walter developed a persistent cough that led to a troubling discovery on his chest x-ray: a suspicious lung nodule that surgical resection eventually confirmed as cancer. He recovered from surgery smoothly and was progressing well when a follow-up CT scan revealed multiple new nodules. He bravely endured subsequent chemotherapy and radiation treatments, although Sarah worried about their efficacy and impact on his declining health.

We met in the office frequently to discuss each new development. Sarah worried that her husband was dying. She agreed to the various treatments but wondered if they were doing more harm than good.

As Walter's condition worsened, the oncologist halted further treatments. Sarah rushed him to the hospital one morning when he couldn't get out of bed. Stepping into Walter's room, I felt a great heaviness overtake me. I found Sarah by his side, holding his hand. She rose to greet me, and as I leaned over Walter, a faint smile crossed his face.

"Doc. I think it's time to call it quits."

My breath caught, and I struggled to respond. As I opened my mouth to speak, I couldn't believe what I found myself saying.

"I'm not ready for you to go!"

Sarah stood beside me, her arm around my shoulder, offering comfort. The memory of Dr. Foster's compassionate act in the ICU flashed through my mind. Perhaps my judgment of him had been too harsh. Sometimes, amid profound loss, it's permissible to lower our defenses and allow moments of vulnerability. There comes a time to transcend roles — doctor, patient, and family — and simply share in the human experience of grief.

Together, we mourned, bound by deep emotional connections, just three individuals navigating the profound loss of a loved one.

Professional distance — the distance healthcare professionals should maintain with their patients to ensure quality care — has its place, but so does intimacy.

A JUDICIOUS MEASURE OF OBTUSENESS

In William Osler's renowned speech delivered as a valedictorian address to the University of Pennsylvania School of Medicine in 1889, he advocates for two specific virtues for graduates to cultivate.[1] The first, "a judicious measure of obtuseness," suggests maintaining an aura of calmness or detachment even in challenging situations, positioning the physician above the fray. The second, "aequanimitas," emphasizes the ability to calmly accept whatever comes next, without descending into emotional hardness.

This balance of obtuseness and aequanimitas remains integral to medical education today, supported by extensive literature advocating for professional distance.[2] This distance safeguards against potential exploitation of the physician-patient power dynamic and maintains the objectivity crucial for medical decision-making.

However, the reality is that this concept of professional distance is more pronounced today than in the past. Just a few decades ago, the landscape of medicine was vastly different, characterized by a greater likelihood of patients knowing, trusting, and respecting their examining physician, who often had insights into their personal lives. Several factors contribute to this shift.

THE DECLINE OF PRIMARY CARE

Medicine once revolved around a singular hub: the primary care physician (PCP). PCPs, including internists, family practitioners, and pediatricians, formed the cornerstone of our healthcare system. They provided continuity of care, often supporting families through generations, which allowed patients to also witness the physician's life milestones like weddings, births, and graduations. In times of personal loss, patients would express condolences or attend funerals — a testament to the deep, personal connections forged.

According to a 2023 report from the Primary Care Collaborative,[3] the number of primary care clinicians has steadily declined due to factors such as burnout, physician shortages, and inadequate investment in the field. Adult PCPs are now estimated to be as little as 25% of the physician workforce.[4] Compare the striking difference from the early 1930s when 87% of private practice physicians were in general care.[5]

Furthermore, there has been a significant decrease in visits to these clinicians. A study published in the *Annals of Family Medicine* highlighted a 20% decline in PCP visits from 2008 to 2015, despite a mere 2.4-minute increase in visit duration.[6] During those 2.4 minutes, on average, 0.3 more diagnoses were addressed.

In essence, our interactions with primary care doctors have become less frequent and more task-oriented, leaving little opportunity for socializing or establishing personal connections.

HOUSE CALLS

Doctors once made house calls, often welcomed into their patients' homes with a seat at the table and a cup of tea. These visits allowed ample time for casual conversation, integrating physicians into the personal intricacies of their patients' lives. The dynamic of the doctor-patient relationship shifted significantly in home settings, where the line between professional and personal barriers blurred slightly.

As a result, physicians typically practiced close to their communities. In those days, neighborhoods were tightly knit, and people often encountered their doctor at church, the grocery store, or local school events. This familiarity extended beyond the medical setting, fostering closer bonds.

However, patient visit demographics underwent profound changes throughout the 20th century. House calls, which constituted 40% of doctor-patient interactions in the 1930s, dwindled to a mere 0.6% by

1980.[7] Consequently, when patients did visit medical offices, they often traveled greater distances. A 2019 Altarum study using data from the Bureau of Labor Statistics' Time Use Survey (2006-2007) revealed that Americans spent an average of 34 minutes commuting to doctor appointments.[8] Based on these trends, it's likely that your doctor today resides miles away from your neighborhood.

THE DIGITAL DISCONNECT

While technology has revolutionized modern healthcare, it has also exacerbated a new digital divide, widening the professional distance between doctors and patients. In many respects, physicians have become captive to our digital tools, prioritizing the care of our computers over that of our patients.

A 2020 study published in the *Annals of Internal Medicine* revealed that physicians spend an average of 16 minutes and 14 seconds per patient encounter on electronic medical records (EMRs).[9] This equates to approximately 45% of a physician's time.[10] In contrast, before the digital era, medical documentation was brief and handwritten, primarily focused on conveying essential information for future patient care.

As Adam Rosen argued in a 2019 *Doximity* opinion piece, we have cultivated a culture akin to distracted driving:[11]

> *"Although providers are mandated to use these systems, it can result in providers being distracted from providing care. I believe a physician caring for a patient while trying to use the EMR is analogous to a distracted driver using a cell phone in traffic. Distracted drivers cause accidents and medical accidents can occur because of distracted providers."*

The issue extends beyond distracted caregiving to include diminished intimacy. This digital barrier inhibits the bidirectional flow of information and empathy, creating not only a physical disconnect but also an emotional disconnect. Research from Northwestern University underscores this, revealing that doctors' eyes are focused on EMRs for about one-third of an average patient visit.[12] This reduced eye contact contrasts starkly with the days of paper charting. Even more surprisingly, patients themselves often find their gaze drawn to the doctor's screen, even when they struggle to comprehend the information displayed.

DISTANCE VERSUS DETACHMENT

Like any professional relationship, boundaries are essential for creating a safe environment and establishing clear roles. In today's modern healthcare practice, where doctors and patients often have no interaction outside of clinical settings, this divide feels more pronounced than ever. Extreme distance can easily verge on detachment, making a doctor's role a delicate balance between remaining detached and engaging.

Various factors have contributed to pushing this balance toward detachment, including the pervasive influence of technology, the widespread burnout among healthcare professionals, and the economic pressures stemming from regulatory demands and competition, particularly from entities like private equity firms. As this trend toward detachment persists, empathy often diminishes.

The Maslach Burnout Inventory, widely used to measure physician burnout, identifies three primary components: emotional exhaustion, depersonalization, and reduced personal accomplishment.[13] Notably, empathy, defined as the ability to understand and share the feelings of others, conflicts with the first two components.

Ultimately, without empathy, genuine intimacy becomes nearly impossible.

EMPATHY IS A PRECURSOR TO INTIMACY

The scientific literature strongly affirms that empathy profoundly enhances the doctor-patient relationship and positively impacts medical outcomes. Research indicates that physician empathy contributes to:[14]

- Enhanced patient satisfaction.
- Improved treatment compliance.
- Better clinical outcomes.
- Increased likelihood of patients practicing self-care.
- Reduced disputes and litigation.
- Improved reimbursement as a result of higher patient experience scores.

- Greater human connection.

While the clinical benefits are evident, it's the emotional benefits that truly make a significant difference. Empathy serves as a crucial foundation for intimacy, which is nonsexual in nature and involves the sharing of deeper thoughts and needs, openness, honesty, and nonjudgmental listening.[15] While complete bidirectional intimacy may not always be appropriate in the exam room, its importance on a broader scale cannot be overstated.

When physicians express empathy and share personal insights in public forums, there is a profound emotional return on investment for patients. While I refrain from discussing my personal needs during a patient's medical emergency, I can and often do share stories and perspectives in public spaces. After years of maintaining a medical blog, I found that my patients developed a biographical understanding of me through our shared experiences, while also gaining emotional insight by reading about my views on various medical issues. They engaged with stories about challenging patients, humbling moments, and critiques of the healthcare system.

STORIES BRIDGE THE INTIMACY GAP

Navigating the dynamics of intimacy between doctors and patients is inherently complex. The traditional role of the physician as the primary seeker of information about patients' personal and medical lives can create a one-sided dynamic. There is not a strict prohibition on doctor-related intimacy within the exam room or hospital, as exemplified by my experiences with patients like Walter and Sarah. I have both laughed and cried with my patients at the appropriate times. We have hugged, held hands, and even high-fived.

The more appropriate and prevalent venue for physician-led intimacy and vulnerability, however, is and should be in public forums. To foster a meaningful version of allyship with those we care for, we must respect the sanctity of the exam room as a space primarily for meeting patients' needs, while also embracing opportunities for public engagement where intimacy can be reciprocated. This approach allows patients not only to learn about our personal backgrounds and societal roles but, more importantly, to understand our values and beliefs. As discussed in the next chapter, storytelling emerges as a powerful tool for achieving this balance.

Exam Room Disclosure

For me, storytelling has unfolded both (sparingly) in the exam room and more expansively in public settings. I have learned to navigate between disclosing appropriate personal insights during clinical encounters and sharing broader narratives outside of them.

I vividly recall the day Lucy, a distraught young mother, walked through my exam room door — an encounter that epitomizes this delicate balance.

Only years later, did I discover just how precarious Lucy's situation had been. When she arrived in my office that day, the unmistakable signs of new motherhood were etched on her face with fatigue. She sank into the chair, exhaling deeply, while her baby and husband waited outside, granting her those brief yet invaluable moments of respite.

As she began detailing her litany of complaints, it became clear that this was a different Lucy from the one I had seen months earlier, before she gave birth. The sparkle in her eyes had dimmed, and her usual vitality had evaporated. In that moment, I instinctively knew that our visit required abandoning the usual playbook. We wouldn't discuss her anemia, allergies, or even the recent thyroid test confirming her medication dosage. Instead, it was apparent that Lucy wasn't in a place to talk at all.

So, I closed my laptop and shared with her the first three months of my own journey with our first child. I spoke of the exhaustion, the loneliness, and the frustration of caring for a newborn who couldn't reciprocate. I didn't diagnose Lucy that day, nor did I submit a bill for the visit. Instead of playing the role of a doctor, I empathized. I conveyed to her that even as a physician — someone expected to have all the answers — I faced similar challenges. I then sent her back out into the world without any specific prescriptions, but with a little more spring in her step.

Life moved forward. I transitioned to a new practice across town, and Lucy and I lost contact. It wasn't until five years later, at an event for our youngest child, that our paths crossed again.

Lucy rushed over and embraced me warmly. She turned to my wife and effusively recounted how I had changed her life that day so many years ago. By reassuring her that her struggles were normal and by sharing my own experiences, I had given her permission to accept her own difficulties. In hindsight, it was a reminder that sometimes the most profound moments in medicine involve simply being human.

Public Disclosure

For years, I wrote publicly about the practice of medicine on a blog called *In My Humble Opinion*. Ironically, my journey into medical blogging began with an interest in artwork. During residency, I ventured into buying and selling art as a side project. My brother, an early 2000s expert in such matters, advised me that better search engine optimization (SEO) could enhance my art business. SEO, a novel concept then, determines how search engines rank websites based on content quality and frequency of updates.

To boost my website's visibility, he urged me to start a blog about art. However, despite my initial optimism, I soon found myself lacking passion for blogging about the art world. One day, I turned to Google and searched "medical blogs," discovering several physician-authored sites dedicated to the practice of medicine.

I was captivated. I stopped writing about artwork and turned my focus to medicine. Over the next decade, I penned about a thousand posts covering everything I wanted to convey about the medical field. Instead of merely imparting knowledge — like how to adjust blood pressure medications — I aimed to reveal who I was. My blog brimmed with impassioned rants, reflections, and my deepest emotions about the profound moments of joy and anguish I encountered daily.

Nearly every blog post held a story — a poignant exploration of the intricate dance between doctor and patient, life and death, and the perpetual clash between selfishness and humanity. I poured my heart and soul onto the page — my blood, sweat, and tears.

It would be years before I realized that my patients had stumbled upon my blog. Occasionally, references in the exam room hinted at their discovery. These posts often sparked deeper conversations, transforming the doctor-patient relationship. My patients began to perceive me differently — not just as a physician, but as a collaborator in their healthcare journey. There was a newfound sense of equality; they had shared their struggles with me in the exam room, and now they read about my challenges online.

It was as if the long-standing paternalism of the doctor-patient had finally faded away.

My shared stories online achieved something that years of face-to-face interactions couldn't: They placed my patients and me in the same arena, fighting a shared battle. For once, they understood they weren't alone in their struggles. Like a phoenix, we faced adversity together, scars and all.

......

For too long, the practice of medicine has operated in a vacuum where patients divulge their most intimate fears and details, receiving little from caregivers in return. This one-sided intimacy has been ingrained in medical tradition, encouraged by heroic and much-praised figures like Osler, who advocated for a professional distance that elevated physicians above emotional entanglements. We have allowed "a judicious measure of obtuseness" and "aequanimitas" to become the standard.

In the past, when medical norms were established, communities were tighter-knit, patients and doctors often lived near each other, fostering personal interactions that underscored the need for professional detachment. However, in today's world, we find ourselves increasingly isolated. Rather than maintaining a balanced distance, we have grown detached, overwhelmed by administrative and technological burdens in caring for patients who are no longer from our immediate communities.

This detachment has eroded empathy and intimacy. While patients continue to share their deepest secrets, physicians often fail to reciprocate in meaningful ways. This distance not only compromises the quality of care but also allows external entities to exploit divisions within the healthcare system.

The remedy lies in rebuilding intimacy. As discussed in the next chapter, the solution is to tell richer, more human stories and to share them openly.

One such story is that of Hunter "Patch" Adams, renowned for his unconventional approach to medicine, emphasizing the healing power of humor and compassion. Through his Gesundheit Institute and advocacy for holistic, patient-centered care, he has inspired a generation of healthcare professionals to prioritize empathy and personal connection in medical practice.

Patch Adams/Tom Shadyac, Robin Williams, Hunter Adams

Hunter "Patch" Adams was notably unimpressed with the movie depicting his early years. He criticized the film, directed by Tom Shadyac and starring Robin Williams, for sacrificing the true importance of his story in favor of commercial appeal, stating it prioritized box office success over authenticity.[16]

Similarly, *Patch Adams* the movie did not garner critical acclaim, receiving a modest rating of just over four out of 10 on Rotten Tomatoes. Critics derided it as overly sentimental. Nevertheless, released in December 1998, the film topped the box office, grossing over $25.2 million in its opening weekend.[17]

Despite its inaccuracies and exaggerated elements, the film shed light on Dr. Adams' remarkable life journey. After battling severe childhood depression and multiple hospitalizations, he proclaimed, "You don't kill yourself, stupid; you make revolution." Adams emerged with a resolve to bring about change through medical school and eventually establish The Gesundheit Institute. According to its website:

> "The Gesundheit Institute, a non-profit healthcare organization, is a project in holistic medical care based on the belief that one cannot separate the health of the individual from the health of the family, the community, the society, and the world. Our mission is to reframe and reclaim the concept of 'hospital'."

Adams believes that laughter, joy, and creativity are integral to the healing process. The portrayal by Tom Shadyac and Robin Williams introduced the public to concepts such as compassion in doctor-patient relationships, the therapeutic value of humor, and the holistic approach to patient care. These ideas contributed significantly to the movement toward patient-centered care, as highlighted in the Institute of Medicine's 2001 report.[18]

CHAPTER TEN.

The Magic of Shared Storytelling

THE PUBLIC IS SELDOM EDUCATED about the trials and tribulations of medical professionals. Patients often lack insight into the challenges doctors face behind the stethoscope. This lack of understanding creates not just an intimacy gap but also an empathy gap.

As discussed in Chapter Nine, the intimacy gap carries significant real-life consequences. Quoting a 2016 *Wall Street Journal* article on storytelling and relationships, historian and literary critic Kari Winter from the University at Buffalo notes:[1]

> *"Stories are profoundly intimate. It is empowering to the teller because they get recognition from the listener. And it is empowering to the listener because it helps them understand the teller."*

Our current healthcare environment has severely damaged the doctor-patient relationship, turning it into a contentious battle where third parties often reap the rewards. Rebuilding intimacy and restoring mutual trust is crucial to ending this exploitation.

We must share our stories. Rebuilding trust will foster allyship — a shared sense of purpose and collective strength to drive meaningful grassroots change. When doctors and patients unite, their combined force will be irresistible.

In this chapter, we will explore storytelling from the perspective of physicians. We will examine how stories manage trauma, build empathy beyond medical circles, and contribute to forging alliances.

But first, allow me to tell you about the day that medicine broke my chief.

THE DAY MEDICINE BROKE MY CHIEF

I was a third-year medical student in the first week of my obstetrics rotation. The obstetrics program was known to be high-pressure, with its residents among the best. Mostly women, they were a hard-core group — smart, efficient, motivated — and they scared the heck out of the medical students.

I remember the day clearly: Not only was I on call, but I was assigned to the chief resident's team. I felt petrified.

We'd started morning rounds as usual, running down the list of patients in labor. Five minutes in, my chief got a "911" page from the ER, located in the next building. This seldom happened, so instead of calling back, we ran downstairs and over to the trauma bay.

We walked into pure chaos. The patient was 27, in her last weeks of pregnancy and bleeding to death. She and her husband had been fighting; apparently, he'd picked up a kitchen knife and stabbed her in the neck.

As the ER physician and the trauma surgeon worked on the woman's neck, my chief readied herself to deliver the baby. She turned to me.

"Quick, get me a sterile gown and a scalpel."

Helping her gown and glove, I saw the other physicians being coated by the blood spurting from the women's neck. She'd been talking when she arrived by ambulance; she wasn't talking anymore.

The nurses were pumping blood into large-bore IVs in both of her arms, but the patient's blood pressure kept dropping. On the fetal monitor, we saw the baby's heart rate starting to dip.

My chief cleared her throat: "Okay, guys, we're gonna lose the baby if we don't do something fast!"

Without taking his eyes from the patient, the trauma surgeon said authoritatively, "We can't. If you cut her, she'll die. Give us a minute."

"It will take a minute-and-a-half to have this baby out," said my chief. She got no answer.

She stood poised over the patient's abdomen, arm raised, scalpel in hand and ready to pounce.

The patient's blood pressure dropped even faster, and the baby's heart rate plummeted.

"It's now or never," said my chief. Then the cardiac monitor began beeping.

"Ventricular fibrillation!" The ER physician grabbed the cardiac paddles and shouted, "Clear!"

With a sweep of his arm, the trauma surgeon moved everyone away from the table, then stepped back … and crashed into my chief. She fell to the floor, extending her arm to avoid slashing anyone with the scalpel.

The electrical shocks, delivered over the course of several minutes, didn't revive the patient. Her wavy cardiac tracing flattened into one long, straight line.

By then it was too late to save the baby. The infant's heart rate had been too low for too long, causing severe, irreversible brain damage. As we listened, the fetal monitor went silent.

The walk back to the obstetrics floor was eerily quiet. I wanted somehow to comfort the chief ... to comfort myself ... but I didn't know how. As we reached the nursing station, she slowly came unwound.

For the first hour, all she wanted to do was talk. She grabbed every resident and nurse who walked by, going over and over what had happened. If only she had disregarded the trauma surgeon, things could have been different....

Then she became intensely quiet. She sat at the table in the middle of the nursing station, her face contorting into a myriad of expressions as she mentally replayed the events. Occasionally she raised her right arm as if wielding the scalpel again.

Finally, she put her head down and started to cry loud, disconcerting sobs. The staff and patients passed to and fro, largely ignoring her. No one seemed to know how to comfort such a strong, accomplished physician in her time of need.

And there I stood, helpless in a sea of sadness and pain.

She cried for what seemed like hours. Then she picked up the phone, made a call, placed her pager on the table, and left the hospital.

A few minutes later, an attending physician came in to replace her, to pick up the pager, and to collect me.

The next day, my chief returned to work. She acted as if nothing had happened. No mention was made of the day before.

She finished the year and is now a well-known attending physician at a prestigious medical center.

I'll always remember that day as the day that medicine broke her, destroyed her innocence. To me, she seemed like a soldier who had witnessed her first death in battle. Would she ever be the same? Or had she lost a sacred part of herself forever?

I feel sure that this is what happened because I remember when medicine broke me one lonely night, watching helplessly as a patient died in the intensive care unit. I'd bet that most of my colleagues have had similar experiences. We rarely talk about them, but you might get some answers if you ask our loved ones.

They would tell you how we changed over the course of our medical training. How one day we came home from work seeming different. How a young, eager, empathic man or woman gradually became angry, frustrated, and cold. How we started out suffering with our patients but ended up suffering from them.

And that's the paradox of medicine. We enter this profession out of a passion to help others. But repeated exposure to the most agonizing situations causes pain that can make us retreat into a shell of cynicism or "clinical objectivity." There, we risk losing the softness, warmth, and caring that sent us into medicine in the first place.

Now, years later, I know that some of us — the lucky ones — recover. For me, the anger and frustration started to reverse 16 years ago with the birth of my son. Gradually, I learned to tend the wounds that medicine had inflicted on me. Now I'm no longer scared of being hurt. Now I can cry *with* my patients, not because of them.

And now I finally feel like the physician I'd always hoped to be: a little more caring, a little more loving, and a little less afraid of what the future will bring.

STORYTELLING AND POST-TRAUMATIC STRESS

There's no way to practice medicine without bearing scars. Almost every physician can recall situations from training or practice that left them with deep feelings of guilt, shame, fear, or sadness. Being a doctor exposes us to life's toughest moments, where we're expected not just to intervene, but to heal. Sometimes it works; other times, it doesn't. And occasionally, our efforts feel more harmful than helpful.

I don't need a study to understand this reality. It was part of my daily experience throughout my medical career, hearing colleagues discuss the haunting moments they try to avoid when left alone in quiet rooms. These emotions, from what I've observed, are nearly universal.

The research regarding post-traumatic stress disorder in physicians varies, suggesting rates ranging from as low as 10%[2] to as high as 31%[3] in the midst of the COVID pandemic. Studies indicate several risk factors, including long working hours, isolation, being female, and pre-existing mental health conditions.

Distressing events, a significant contributor to PTSD, are alarmingly prevalent, with nearly 80% of doctors reporting at least one in the past year.[4] Moreover, more than two-thirds of providers involved in adverse clinical events experience troubling memories, anxiety, anger, remorse, and distress, according to recent studies.[5]

For me, the solution to my trauma-induced depression and anxiety was storytelling. Publishing my experience in *Pulse: Voices from the Heart of Medicine*[6] allowed me to finally release the pain and hurt I had carried. I found solace in knowing I was not alone in this journey.

Narrative exposure therapy, originally developed for refugees who endured torture and hardships, is a treatment approach for trauma disorders like PTSD where sufferers create a narrative of traumatic life events. Proven effective in treating PTSD,[7] it involves creating a chronological history of the traumatic experience, incorporating positive elements, and revisiting and refining the narrative to achieve understanding and acceptance of the trauma.

The power of storytelling is further amplified when shared between doctors and patients. In June 2022, Drs. Mariam Alam and Caitlin Crimp received a grant from the Accreditation Council for Graduate Medical Education's (ACGME) Back to Bedside program. Their collaborative project, "Mitigating Bias and Burnout Through Patient-Centered Narrative Medicine," developed a narrative medicine curriculum for dermatology residents. This initiative brought panels of patients and caregivers together to foster empathy and understanding:[8]

> *"During each Narrative Medicine Patient Panel, residents are asked to read and critically analyze a piece of literature, poem or article related to the panel topic. Residents are encouraged to ask patients questions, and afterward are asked to write a brief self-reflection in response to a prompt, discussing what they learned and their thoughts, feelings and reactions to the panelists."*

These panels not only provided therapeutic benefits for patients but also fostered a newfound sense of empathy and compassion among participating physicians. Moreover, they inspired clinicians to engage in their own reflective writing, focusing on challenging patient interactions.

When clinicians and patients collaborate in writing, the benefits extend to everyone involved. Researchers from Rosalind Franklin University and Advocate Children's Hospital introduced the 'Three-Minute Mental Makeover (3MMM), an uncomplicated but research-backed journaling technique that may significantly reduce stress with lasting effects. Practitioners and patients/families used a structured script to write simultaneously. They then shared their responses, with presurvey and postsurvey data analyzed using nonparametric tests.[9]

Key findings included:

- At baseline, all patients, family members, and practitioners reported experiencing one or more symptoms of stress.
- After engaging in the 3MMM activity, patients/family members and practitioners reported reduced stress compared to baseline.
- Practitioners noted a significant improvement in communication skills.
- Despite only 35% of patients/families having used writing or journaling previously, 88% found the 3MMM activity helpful.

The mutual exchange of stories proved beneficial for everyone involved, enhancing communication and reducing stress levels among practitioners and patients alike.

THE EMPATHY GAP

It's not just patients who crave understanding; physicians often grapple with the perception that the public doesn't grasp the trauma and challenges inherent in their profession. While medical trainees are immersed in a rigorous, trial-by-fire introduction to clinical practice, the general public remains largely shielded from the daily stresses of doctors. This isolation has contributed to a widespread sense of loneliness for physicians.

In a 2018 survey conducted by Athena Health of nearly 1,400 practicing physicians, 25% reported feeling isolated in their professional lives at least once a week, with 6% experiencing daily isolation.[10]

Despite interacting with numerous patients throughout the day, there remains a professional disconnect. Patients rarely comprehend the emotional realities of being a doctor. The necessary barrier between practitioner and patient exists to uphold professionalism and expertise, and safeguard the public from the more distressing aspects of our caregiving roles. My friends and family outside of medicine have little desire to hear about the sights, sounds, and odors of caring for dying patients. They chose different paths for valid reasons, opting not to enter the medical field or specialize in hospice care.

Yet, in my own experience, sharing these realities through storytelling can foster a deeper and more engaged relationship between doctors and patients. While we frequently emphasize the importance of the patient narrative and train on how to make patients feel heard, we often overlook the doctor's own need to feel heard. In many ways, we've been deprived of the opportunity to share our own narrative, to tell our stories.

We've also been deprived of having our empathy reciprocated. While there may be a one-way intimacy gap between doctors and patients, there certainly exists an empathy gap that flows in the opposite direction. Part of the issue is that the average patient cannot fathom the challenges of being a caregiver. They have not experienced the sleep deprivation, split-second decisions, or profound guilt that accompanies each loss. They don't comprehend the constant self-doubt, the complex nuances involved in medical decision-making, or the erosion of autonomy and the pressures of compliance.

They don't know because we haven't told them. As doctors, we excel at sharing our medical knowledge with patients but often fail to convey who we are as individuals. How can the public empathize with us when they do not understand our struggles? We have so rigidly defined ourselves through professionalism and by maintaining a professional distance that we have become invisible.

We can't be seen for who we are.

Storytelling has the power to bridge these gaps. It is the antidote to distance. By sharing our stories, we can close both the intimacy and empathy gaps. We will reveal what lies deepest within us, and in doing so, we will not only share ourselves but also receive the empathy that our profession desperately needs.

It's about giving and receiving. Telling and listening. Working toward the ultimate goal of intimacy. It's about forging alliances.

ALLYSHIP REDEFINED

We often discuss allyship in the context of diversity, equity, and inclusion. Allyship entails actions, behaviors, and practices where leaders support, amplify, and advocate for others, particularly those who do not share the same social identities.[11] In the realm of healthcare, I propose redefining allyship to focus on the differing social identities of doctors (caregivers) and patients, rather than on racial or gender disparities.

For too long, the healthcare system and its third-party entities have sought to drive a wedge between us. In any community, whether corporate or otherwise, stakeholders are defined as those who are affected by the community or its operations — including employees, customers, suppliers, local communities, environmental groups, governmental bodies, and more.[12] Within the United States healthcare system, I argue for prioritizing doctors (and other caregivers) and patients over these extractive third parties.

Yet, to bridge the divide and unite these major stakeholders — who are more divided than ever — we need a mechanism to rebuild allyship. Storytelling serves as a critical strategy. Storytelling has several profound ways of bringing stakeholders together:[13]

1. Stories evoke profound emotions. Nearly every significant medical encounter is laden with intense emotion. When doctors share their stories, they reveal that patients aren't alone in experiencing deep feelings. There's a shared sense of fear, anxiety, joy, and triumph. While these emotions have often remained isolated, storytelling offers a path to connect them in the future.
2. Stories foster relatability. Doctors and patients inherently view our medical system from distinct perspectives. While doctors may eventually become patients, most patients won't experience being physicians. Through shared storytelling, common themes, struggles, and challenges emerge, despite differing details.
3. Stories communicate values and vision. Amid the complexities of medical encounters, it can be easy to lose sight of the core values each party brings to the table. Medicine is intricate, and nuances can get lost in the process. Storytelling reminds stakeholders that shared values and goals exist.

4. Stories simplify intricate concepts. Disease processes and medical terminology can seem incomprehensible to those outside the field. Storytelling elucidates these complexities and sheds light on deeper, nuanced truths.
5. Stories create lasting impressions. Stories are memorable. We recall moments when doctors shared their personal reality, or when patients opened up about their childhood fears and concerns. These narratives linger, deepening our understanding and compassion for one another.

······

In the early 2000s, I began on an impulse to write about medicine. What started as a way to tell my stories evolved into a therapeutic exchange with my past and my patients. Through this process, I became acutely aware of the profound intimacy gap between doctors and patients. Using storytelling, I could bridge this gap by sharing the gifts of my patients' bodies and souls through my narratives. This is the transformative power of shared storytelling.

As opposed to lining up on opposite sides of the football field, we found ourselves collaborating as primary stakeholders in our healthcare system. It was us against the world. My ability to deeply listen to and understand my patients' narratives, and subsequently write about medicine and the doctor-patient relationship, has been part of a broader movement that has been gaining momentum over the decades. This movement is known as *narrative medicine* and one of its main supporters is a doctor named Rita Charon.

Narrative Medicine: Honoring the Stories of Illness/ Rita Charon

Rita Charon is a pioneering figure and authority in the burgeoning field of narrative medicine. She defines narrative medicine as:[14]

> *"Medicine practiced with the competence to recognize, absorb, interpret, and be moved by the stories of illness. By placing events in temporal order, with beginnings, middles, and ends, and by establishing connections among things using metaphor and figural language,*

narrative medicine helps doctors to recognize patients and diseases, convey knowledge, accompany patients through the ordeals of illness — and ultimately lead to more humane, ethical, and effective health care."

Narrative competence, the ability to navigate these narratives, allows physicians to engage with four central narrative situations in medicine:

- Physician and patient
- Physician and self
- Physician and colleagues
- Physicians and society

Exploring these narratives enables physicians to empathize with their patients during illness, acknowledge their own personal journeys, connect with the experiences of fellow caregivers, and initiate dialogues with the public about healthcare. As Charon puts it, "by bridging the divides that separate physicians from patients, themselves, colleagues, and society, narrative medicine offers fresh opportunities for respectful, empathic, and nourishing medical care."

Charon's teachings and her seminal book have become the definitive voice of the narrative medicine movement. Both aspiring and seasoned physicians increasingly use the power of storytelling alongside medical practice to better address the significant gaps present in modern medicine today.

And because of it, medicine has become more humane — more human-centered.

TEN WAYS PHYSICIANS SHARE PATIENT-CENTERED STORIES

Here's a list of 10 places where doctors can and should share patient stories, along with brief descriptions:

1. **Medical Conferences and Grand Rounds:** Doctors often present patient cases during medical conferences and grand rounds to educate colleagues on complex diagnoses, treatment challenges, and clinical outcomes.
2. **Medical Journals and Case Reports:** Published case reports in medical journals provide detailed accounts of unique or noteworthy patient cases, contributing to medical literature and education.
3. **Blogs and Personal Websites:** Many doctors maintain blogs or personal websites where they share anonymized patient stories to

illustrate medical principles, ethical dilemmas, or personal reflections.

4. **Social Media:** Platforms like X, Facebook, and Instagram allow doctors to share patient stories in a more public and accessible format, often with educational or advocacy purposes.
5. **Podcasts:** Medical podcasts frequently feature doctors discussing patient cases, treatment approaches, and clinical insights, reaching a broad audience of healthcare professionals and the public.
6. **Medical Education and Training Programs:** Within medical schools, residency programs, and continuing medical education (CME) courses, instructors use patient stories to teach students about diagnosis, treatment planning, and patient care.
7. **Ethics Committees and Case Discussions:** Hospitals and healthcare institutions convene ethics committees where doctors present anonymized patient cases to discuss ethical dilemmas, patient rights, and care decisions.
8. **Healthcare Quality Improvement Initiatives:** In efforts to improve healthcare quality, doctors share patient stories in quality improvement projects to identify systemic issues, enhance patient safety, and optimize care processes.
9. **Public Speaking Engagements:** Doctors often speak at public events, community forums, or TED-style talks, using patient stories to highlight healthcare challenges, promote awareness, and advocate for policy changes.
10. **Books and Memoirs:** Some doctors write books or memoirs that include patient stories to convey personal experiences, medical insights, and the emotional impact of patient care on their professional lives.

Each of these platforms serves different purposes, from medical education and advocacy to ethical reflection and public awareness, while respecting patient confidentiality and privacy regulations.

CHAPTER ELEVEN.

How To Share Our Stories in Real Time

WHILE SHARED STORYTELLING MAY SEEM appealing in theory, its appropriateness in many medical settings is debatable. When patients seek solace in a doctor's office, the last thing they want is to hear a clinician recounting their own worries and troubles.

The examination room has historically served — and should continue to serve — as a sanctuary of safety for weary patients. However, this doesn't imply that the medical community cannot express itself through other channels. For decades, we've used traditional and social media to disseminate our knowledge. It's time to use these platforms to also reveal who we are. We need open, real-time dialogues about our experiences — the highs and lows, fears and triumphs. Public discussions on medical malpractice and clinical errors are crucial. Healthcare providers should have a platform to share their victories and setbacks.

Re-establishing meaningful communication channels is essential, but we must also prioritize patient confidentiality and respect. Just as we wouldn't divulge personal stories in a crowded elevator, we shouldn't disclose identifiable medical details on public platforms like Facebook or Instagram.

This chapter will explore best practices for safely and honestly sharing stories in the digital age, a practice that can be particularly nuanced and challenging, as illustrated by the following example.

HIDDEN DEPTHS

I was captivated by the reason Annie couldn't proceed with the MRI. Despite knowing her for over a decade, I had never heard about the day her childhood home burned down — how she had been trapped under her bed, convinced at five years old that she wouldn't survive.

She didn't die. Instead, she recalls the strong forearms of the fireman who rescued her, carrying her through flames to safety. While her body survived, her fear of confined spaces persisted throughout her life.

This fear rarely surfaced in ordinary circumstances, but when she was placed inside the MRI machine and the relentless clunking commenced, the confined space triggered a panic. She pounded against the tube, pleading to be freed.

It wasn't until a week later in my office that Annie could articulate her ordeal. We discussed her post-traumatic stress and whether she had sought treatment for it. Together, we opted for an alternative method to obtain the necessary diagnostic information. That day, we both left the exam room with a deeper understanding of Annie's needs.

A year later, I decided to write a blog post on my public blog about Annie's experience. In the story, however, Annie became Jake, the MRI became a CPAP machine, and the house fire transformed into an incident where Jake was trapped as a rescue worker in a coal mine collapse. I wrote the story and, honestly, didn't think much about it afterward.

Yet, Annie had read the story on my blog and brought it up at our next visit. Her words caught me off guard:

"I can't imagine going through something so traumatic!"

Surprisingly, she hadn't recognized herself in the story. It was a realization that shaped my approach whenever I share a patient's story publicly, whether with their explicit permission or not.

NARRATIVE NUANCE

Throughout this book, I've championed the concept of shared storytelling, yet we must carefully consider the ethical implications of recounting patient anecdotes. Patient privacy rights are paramount under regulations like HIPAA, which define protected health information broadly, encompassing identifiable details such as names, health conditions, treatments, and personal data. Sharing such information unequivocally breaches privacy.

The larger quandary revolves around what constitutes identifiable information. Can anonymity alone suffice? What if details are altered to obscure identification, as I did in recounting Annie's story, changing even significant details like gender or medical condition? As we explore later in this chapter, thoughtful consideration should enable us to honor patient privacy while conveying the profound insights gained from shared experiences.

There is also a subtler concern regarding narrative dynamics. As narrators, there's a tendency to adopt a paternalistic stance toward our subjects, potentially compromising the dignity and respect they deserve. As articulated by sociologist Arthur Frank, whose expertise spans narrative ethics, narrative medicine, and narrative therapy:[1]

> *"What we need instead is narrative nuance. We need to understand how to tell respectful stories in which the patients are fully acknowledged fellow participants, not one-dimensional objects of a knowing gaze. The problem is not narration itself but a particular version of narrational privilege, and getting rid of that would have benefits far beyond practices of writing case studies."*

Understanding this narrative privilege allows us to move past the pronouns of *yours* and *mine* and more comfortably into telling *our* story. These narratives belong jointly to the narrator and the subject, to both doctor and patient. Narrative nuance underscores the shared nature of storytelling — not just the act of recounting in each other's company but the mutual ownership of the narrative itself.

These are our stories!

"What Happened Truth"

Ultimately, any writer weaving narratives about patients faces a crucial decision between portraying "story truth" and adhering strictly to "what happened truth," a distinction Tim O'Brien famously elucidates by pointing to the difference that occurs with merging and deidentifying stories versus sticking to the actual facts of the case.[2]

"What happened truth," in its purest form, necessitates seeking consent directly from the patient or story subject. As Danielle Ofri underscores in her piece for the *Huffington Post*, patients entrust us with their vulnerabilities and pain, necessitating that their interests be prioritized ethically.[3] Should a story later warrant a broader audience, obtaining consent becomes an imperative ethical step.

In today's landscape, consent forms are increasingly commonplace, driven by marketing and promotional activities. Practitioners, hospital systems, and online platforms frequently solicit testimonials that may include significant medical details. These consent forms typically include:

- An authorization to use a story/photo/or video.
- A listing of where the info is expected to appear.
- An acknowledgment of any payment or whether the story will be used for commercial purposes.
- An acknowledgment that the story may disclose protected health information.
- A protocol for revoking permission to use the story (if possible).

Adhering to these guidelines allows medical professionals to ethically secure permission, ensuring accurate depiction while possibly disclosing protected information. Providing subjects an opportunity to review the material before publication further respects their autonomy.

"Story Truth"

Much of my writing about medicine over the years has predominantly embraced what's known as "story truth." This style of storytelling hinges on thematic integrity while altering specific details to safeguard the protagonist's identity or enhance narrative coherence. While these modifications uphold thematic truth, the standards for such practices vary. Some advocate the elevator rule — never disclose in writing what you wouldn't say aloud in a hospital elevator. Personally, I adhere to a stricter standard: If the protagonist or their close associates cannot identify the character in the story, then the disguise is successful.

Regrettably, the guidelines governing privacy and medical narratives remain ambiguous. Authors wield considerable discretion in disguising identities and exercising creative license. However, overindulgence in creative liberty risks eroding trust between storyteller and audience. Balancing the need for discretion with preserving the essential truths of a narrative demands the narrative nuance I highlighted earlier. It's a delicate balance, but the potential rewards are substantial.

The Medium

We've devoted considerable discussion to the ethics and methods of storytelling, but up to this point, we've neglected to address where these stories are shared. With the rise of social media, podcasts, and platforms like TED Talks and The Moth, we've moved away from traditional mediums such as books and articles. This shift has had both positive and negative impacts.

On the positive side, these platforms have lowered barriers to entry, making it easy for almost anyone to start a blog, launch a podcast, or share thoughts on platforms like Instagram and TikTok. This accessibility has democratized medical publishing, offering a voice to anyone with a story to tell. While liberating for content creators seeking an audience, it also means there's little regulation of storytelling on the internet.

Conversely, the downside is that deeply personal information can quickly become public fodder. Protected health information can be disseminated globally in an instant. While the internet excels at spreading positive messages, this same capability can inadvertently harm patients. A mishandled story can persist online indefinitely, serving as a constant reminder of trauma, misfortune, or embarrassment for the patient.

Our intent as healthcare providers is to help, not inadvertently cause harm. This remains an area where safety and guidelines need to thoughtfully be developed on an ongoing basis.

Narrative Empathy

Ultimately, our mission to support patients, foster allyship, and enhance care hinges on a broader narrative among physicians. While we delve into stories that explore the complexities of caregiving — its decisions and burdens — when patient narratives enter the discussion, physician writers must be acutely attuned to the tone and perspective of their storytelling.

There's a tendency to position oneself as the omniscient narrator, treating characters in the story as subjects to be analyzed, and perhaps manipulated, for the storyteller's benefit. While effective in fiction, medical writing demands a more rigorous approach: not only representing caregivers but also authentically conveying the patient's experience.

Narration should naturally reflect shared experiences and empathetic nuance. As physicians, we hold our patients' stories with great responsibility. This entails going beyond mere actions or our interpretations, and instead, articulating their narratives in alignment with their voices.

As adept clinicians and storytellers, we excel at deciphering the narratives of individuals navigating illness and health. If our aim is allyship, we must move beyond mere depiction to true advocacy — we must speak *for* them and not just *of* them. What I advocate for here transcends mere narrative finesse; it embodies what I call narrative empathy. Through these stories, we should aim to enable our readers to step into the shoes of those we care for.

Our role is that of a conduit. We receive our patients' stories, weaving together coherence and detail, adding our insights while preserving their essence intact. These are the lived experiences of others entrusted to us, allowing us to extract meaning, establish connections, and foster empathy and understanding.

This demands an exquisite respect and clarity in our portrayal of subjects. Our tone should reflect reverence, gratitude, and awe. In our narratives, our patients are the teachers, and we the eager learners.

PHYSICIAN STORYTELLERS THROUGH THE AGES

The roster of physician storytellers is extensive, well-rooted, and ever-expanding. Surprisingly, some historical figures gained more renown for their writing than their medical deeds. Going back as far as medieval times, figures such as the philosopher and physician Maimonides stand out. Maimonides not only chronicled medical conditions such as asthma, diabetes, hepatitis, and pneumonia but also stressed the importance of moderation and healthy living. His writings transcended his time, influencing both medicine and philosophy for centuries.[4]

John Locke, a 17th-century English philosopher and physician, is celebrated as one of the most influential thinkers of the Enlightenment era, often hailed as the "father of liberalism."[5] In the 18th century, luminaries like John Keats, Edward Jenner, Tobias George Smollett, Anton Chekov, Sir Arthur Conan Doyle, and Oliver Wendell Holmes rose to prominence. In the 19th century, figures such as W. Somerset Maugham, Sir William Osler, and William Carlos Williams were celebrated for their contributions.

Not to be outdone, the 20th and 21st centuries have witnessed the emergence of notable medical writers such as Oliver Sacks and Atul Gawande. *When Breath Becomes Air*, the poignant memoir by the late neurosurgeon Paul Kalanithi, was published in 2016 and remained on the *New York Times* nonfiction bestseller list for 68 weeks.

Books, however, have taken a backseat to more contemporary forms of communication in the 21st century. TEDMED, an annual conference focused on health and medicine, has gained prominence. While in-person attendance is limited by available space, the talks are widely accessible via YouTube, reaching millions. Medical blogs continue to thrive, with long-standing favorites like Dr. Kevin Pho's *KevinMD* blog,[6] which has been a cornerstone since the early 2000s.

Doctors have also embraced audio mediums for storytelling. The proliferation of medical podcasts exemplifies this trend, with shows like *The Nocturnists* podcast by Dr. Emily Silverman serving as a vibrant platform where healthcare workers celebrate their humanity through compelling narratives.[7]

My Decades of Writing about Medicine

One of my earliest forays into writing about medicine occurred during my first year of medical school, when I served as a hospice volunteer. Amid the profound experiences of grief, sorrow, and occasional wonder, I penned a poem titled "I Am the Father" (included at the end of this chapter), which explores the myriad roles played out at the bedside of a dying patient. The impact was immediate: Sharing this poem with medical staff and patients' families forged a new intimacy. Being able to empathize with the perspectives of the patient, family members, chaplain, and ultimately the doctor enabled me to articulate the complex, poignant, and often uplifting narratives woven around the journey through life's final moments.

Writing became a significant outlet during my medical school and residency years, with numerous poems and reflections eventually finding their way into medical journals and culminating in my own chapbook of poetry. This passion for expression led me into the realm of blogging. Initially focused on the art world, my interests soon expanded to include medical blogging, beginning in 2004 with *In My Humble Opinion*.[8] Over the next decade, I maintained a prolific output, sometimes posting daily, and even compiled selected blog entries into two anthologies spanning medical and nonmedical narratives.

Simultaneously, I joined a medical speaker's bureau, where I brought these stories to life in discussions on topics ranging from the doctor-patient relationship to hospice care and the evolving role of social media in healthcare. Writing about medicine and sharing my experiences opened doors to speaking engagements at national and international conferences, participation on advisory panels for corporations, and a means to process the emotional challenges many physicians face.

Above all, becoming a doctor storyteller transformed my relationship with patients in ways that traditional doctoring had not. While as a physician, I had been their adviser and advocate, translating the complexities of the human body, storytelling allowed me to journey alongside them as a companion. We forged bonds as fellow travelers, sharing the hidden joys and hardships of our shared path. We became allies. We became intimate confidants.

......

Few experiences match the profoundness of being at the bedside with a dying patient and their family. As physicians, these moments are rare, shifting our focus from active intervention to providing comfort and dignity. Our role becomes one of vigilance in alleviating suffering while allowing nature to take its course quietly and with dignity and grace.

Many physicians have captured their reflections on death, seeking to convey not just the pain but also the enduring human spirit that emerges during life's final season. Caring for the dying remains one of the few arenas where professional distance can yield to emotional engagement. In hospice care, caregivers are encouraged to empathize deeply with patients and families, standing together in shared humanity.

Yet, when we as physicians recount these experiences, we must tread carefully not to overshadow the patient's own voice. Amid our reflections and emotions, it's easy to unintentionally reduce the dying to mere subjects of our narratives rather than honoring their full humanity.

I penned the poem "I Am the Father" to articulate the profound emotions of being present with a dying patient and their loved ones. This poem isn't meant to evoke sentimentality but to offer a perspective from the doctor's lens, recognizing that each narrator brings a unique voice and viewpoint. Through these narratives, we come to understand our interconnectedness in both profound and challenging ways.

In these moments, we realize that our lives intertwine — doctors, patients, and family members. For those who haven't experienced these situations firsthand, poems and stories offer a glimpse into the depths of these human experiences.

I Am the Father/Jordan Grumet (As published in Primary Care)[9]

I am the father and have come to die, help me go in peace:

I am the doctor and I have known you for many years. The day I told you the diagnosis I watched you break down and cry right there in my office. I held your hand and told you everything would be okay but I didn't know how. We fought together as a team. My patient, my fellow soldier in a losing battle I've done all I can. I hold your hands not only to comfort you but also to reframe what once I believed were hands only capable of healing. Before you I never realized that "to do no harm" meant admitting that the most sanctified of holy arts is often imperfect and helpless. I want to bring you peace. I yearn to erase the unfathomable gulf between two hearts, one of which will soon die and the other remains.

I am the father and have come to die, help me go in peace:

I am the wife and my heart is breaking with your every labored breath. When we said at the dawn of our voyage "till death do us part" I had no idea that the dusky shore was following so close beyond the horizon. Through the years of supporting you and giving you strength I developed an identity intimately touched by your life. How easy it was to think that you were the one who needed me. As I see the life slowly fade from your body I am aware of losing a wonderful part of myself. The light of my life is dimming and I am afraid of the dark. You were my constant companion through the years. We could win any battle as long as we fought together. The father of my children, the laughter behind my smile; I'm not ready for you to go. You ask for peace but I don't know how to quiet the torment engulfing my heart. I do not feel peace. I want to be strong but it takes all my energy to keep from breaking down. I want to shake you with all my might and yell at you for leaving me behind. I want to pick you up and cradle you in my arms and let my love heal you. Could my love heal you?

I am the father and have come to die, help me go in peace:

I am the son and also search for peace. Through all those years you took care of me and led my way. You fed my mind, heart, and soul as readily as my body. You sculpted me in the image of your god, passing on everything in your heart that was most precious. There was no problem you couldn't solve for me. There was nothing you weren't willing to give. When disease overcame you I wrongly felt I could repay your never ending love. I sit by your side for endless hours, cleaning you, feeding you, anticipating your needs. I am now the father, you are now the son. I have lost my job, I am losing my family. I thought I was strong enough to care for you. I thought I could singlehandedly bear the weight of the world. I'm afraid this dreaded disease is taking my life as well as yours. I can't do this anymore. How can one in search of life submerge himself in death?

I am the father and have come to die, help me go in peace:

I am the daughter and I haven't seen you in ten years. As a child your presence itself was enough to make me hate you. I was never good enough; I never did the right thing. When I became an adult I ran as far away as possible. I built a life of my own. One in which you couldn't invade. I cut you out with a sneer, always knowing deep down inside that it hurt; that one day I would have to address my feelings. Well, the day is now. Before I figured that I had more time. That if I put it off today there would always be tomorrow. Days turned into months, months into years, and before I knew it a decade passed. I am aware that no story is truly one-sided and I regret never taking the time to listen to yours. I am sorry that you are going to die. Between you and me, the time for peace has come.

I am the father and have come to die and now I have found peace:

Under the weight of my sickly body my soul has emerged lucid and strong. My fear of death has been replaced with the wish that I may die with all the hope and dignity that I struggled to live life. I have replayed the story of my life over and over in my mind. I accept it as a battle littered with majestic happiness as well as painful sorrow. I have known the greatest love and the greatest hurt. I know I have found peace because inwardly I am very thankful, to have been a part of this wonderful dance we call life. Tomorrow when the doctor comes I will thank him for all he has done. I will tell my son to go home and take care of his family. The peace that he is looking for can only be found in his children. I will forgive my daughter and ask for her forgiveness. I will tell her that no matter how bad things were between us I always loved her. And lastly, I will hold my wife in my arms and cry like the day she agreed to marry me. And then I will give up this fight and die the victor.

BEST PRACTICES FOR MEDICAL STORYTELLING

When doctors decide to share patient stories publicly, whether in writing, speaking engagements, or through media, it's crucial to consider appropriate ethical and professional guidelines to protect patient confidentiality, respect privacy, and uphold trust. Here are some best practices:

Obtain Informed Consent. When possible, seek explicit permission from the patient (or their legally authorized representative) before sharing any details about their medical history, condition, or personal experiences. Ensure the patient understands how their story will be used, where it will be shared, and any potential risks.

Anonymize and De-identify. If obtaining explicit consent is not feasible or if the patient prefers anonymity, ensure all identifying details are removed or altered to prevent identification. Change names, locations, ages, and any other specifics that could lead to the patient's identification.

Focus on Generalized and Educational Content. When discussing patient stories, focus on general medical conditions, experiences, or scenarios that are educational and relatable without divulging specific details that could lead to patient identification. Emphasize broader themes and lessons learned rather than individual cases.

Maintain Confidentiality. Never disclose patient information in public forums, social media, or any unsecured platforms. Avoid using patient-specific details, medical records, images, or videos without explicit permission, even in educational contexts.

Use Composite Cases. When illustrating medical cases, consider using composite cases where details from multiple patients are combined to represent a generalized scenario. This helps in protecting individual patient privacy while still conveying educational content.

Educate and Sensitize. Educate colleagues, students, and the public about the importance of patient confidentiality and privacy. Foster an environment where respect for patient stories and confidentiality is prioritized.

Seek Guidance and Policies. Refer to institutional policies, professional guidelines (e.g., from medical boards or associations), and legal requirements regarding patient privacy and confidentiality. Stay updated on ethical standards and best practices in medical storytelling.

Respect Cultural Sensitivities. Consider cultural, religious, and social sensitivities when sharing patient stories. Respect diverse perspectives and avoid stereotypes or stigmatizing language that could harm patients or their communities.

Monitor Impact and Feedback. Be mindful of the potential impact of sharing patient stories on patients, families, and the community. Monitor feedback and responses to ensure stories are shared responsibly and ethically.

Reflect and Evaluate. Regularly reflect on your storytelling practices and evaluate their impact on patient care, trust, and professional ethics. Continuously strive to improve communication and ethical standards in medical storytelling.

By following these best practices, doctors can responsibly share patient stories to educate, advocate, and raise awareness while maintaining patient confidentiality, trust, and respect.

CHAPTER TWELVE.

How Stories Become Reality: Transforming Our Healthcare System

THE INPATIENT PAVILION AND ADMINISTRATIVE CENTER where I began my hospice career holds a cherished place in my heart. I started consulting with this hospice around 2010 when they were one of the largest providers in the area, often caring for up to 1,500 patients daily.

The pavilion was always bustling with activity. There were numerous employees, multiple team meetings, several conference rooms, and sometimes up to 15 patients in the specialized inpatient hospice unit. The facility was led by a physician and passionate advocate for hospice and palliative care. She fostered an environment centered on patients, combining academic medicine with ongoing education and advocacy.

In addition to doctors and nurses, certified nursing assistants, music therapists, and massage practitioners filled the halls. Laughter echoed, team huddles were commonplace, and birthdays and anniversaries were joyfully celebrated. Every patient's passing was honored with music that played throughout the building, and staff often gathered to witness patients' families leaving the facility for the last time.

As a not-for-profit organization, the hospice relied not only on Medicare and insurance billing but also heavily on community donations. It was clear that no one entered this field for financial gain; physicians, nurses, and administrators received modest salaries, driven by a shared commitment rather than monetary rewards.

As the years passed, changes inevitably swept through. Faced with fierce competition from newly acquired hospitals, private hospices, and mounting legislative demands, this esteemed hospice was compelled to merge with two others in the area.

This new conglomerate, born of both business acumen and clinical expertise, evolved over time. Emphasis shifted to maximizing profits, sidelining extras like massage therapists. The corporate leadership, once intertwined with clinical care, gradually distanced itself; senior physicians departed as the organization's priorities shifted. Gone were the birthday celebrations, and the camaraderie among team members dwindled.

A series of misfortunes struck. A misguided decision by the corporate team to acquire a home health practice and subsequent compliance fines stemming from a merger mishap dealt severe blows to the once-thriving hospice.

Faced with a stark choice of survival or demise, the hospice succumbed. It was sold to a private equity firm specializing in distressed hospices, signaling a shift to a more profit-driven model. While employees retained their jobs, benefits were slashed, hours extended, and a new operational framework imposed.

The hospice pavilion, originally erected with generous community donations, once teeming with life and community engagement, was downsized and eventually shuttered to align with corporate strategies.

Years later, it remains empty. Passing by occasionally on my way to run errands, I reflect on the profound impact that building had on countless lives — patients spending their final days there and the employees who once formed a vibrant, caring community.

Undoubtedly, it was a pavilion built on love and dismantled by corporate greed.

If we want our healthcare system to change, we are going to have to fight for it. Stopping the ruthless destruction of what love has built demands a concerted effort to eradicate the greed that pervades our cherished healthcare institutions. The legislative process, marred by entrenched interests, has repeatedly proven inadequate on its own.

What's imperative now is a revolution — a spark that ignites transformative action. Yet, upon closer inspection, these sparks have always been present, awaiting our collective resolve to stoke their flames. It's time to amplify our stories, to resonate with purpose and impact.

The profound impact of shared storytelling on healthcare practices and costs is well-documented globally, notably exemplified by Dr. A.J. Cronin's narrative and its pivotal role in shaping England's nationalized health service. This narrative, however, is just one of many.

Numerous contemporary examples underscore the transformative power of shared stories in modern medicine. Sherwin Newland's 2001

Ted Talk, "How Electroshock Therapy Changed Me," resonated widely, dispelling myths perpetuated by popular culture about this critical treatment modality.

Similarly, Atul Gawande's 2014 book, *Being Mortal,* intertwined personal and patient stories to critique end-of-life care, catalyzing widespread awareness of systemic shortcomings.

In this chapter, we delve into these narratives, illustrating how storytelling catalyzes enduring change and enriches our community's health discourse.

A UNIVERSALLY BELOVED DOCTOR

The United Kingdom's National Health Service (NHS) is frequently praised as a step in the right direction toward what healthcare could resemble in the United States. Established in 1948, it has evolved into the world's largest publicly funded health program.[1] Healthcare spending in the United Kingdom as a percentage of GDP has risen steadily since 1990, from 5.1% to 11.3% by 2022.[2] In contrast, the United States spent 17.3% of its GDP on healthcare in the same year.[3] Public funding covers a substantial 79.5% of health expenditure in the United Kingdom, with out-of-pocket expenses relatively low at 17% (2019). Private medical insurance typically fills gaps in NHS coverage or provides faster access to services.[4] Despite recent declines in public satisfaction, support for the NHS's fundamental principles remains robust.[5]

The NHS, however, is a relatively recent initiative that faced significant challenges before its establishment. According to *Historic UK,* the movement for a nationalized health service was driven by dedicated individuals seeking to reform the existing system. This effort began in the early 1900s, catalyzed by a government report from noted socialist Beatrice Webb.[6] Webb argued convincingly for a new healthcare system to replace the antiquated Poor Law, which had its roots in the Victorian-era workhouses. Dr. Benjamin Moore, a physician from Liverpool, notably penned "The Dawn of the Health Age" in 1911, likely one of the earliest uses of the phrase "National Health Service."[7] However, public support for the idea fluctuated during the interwar period between World War I and World War II.

And then a pivotal transformation occurred. As documented by *Historic UK*:[6]

> *"Further momentum was gained when Dr. A.J. Cronin's novel* The Citadel *was published in 1937 and proved to be highly controversial for its criticism of the inadequacies and failures of healthcare. The book was based on a story about a doctor from a small Welsh mining village who climbed the ranks to become a doctor in London. Cronin had observed the medical scene greatly and the book prompted new ideas about medicine and ethics, inspiring to some extent the NHS and the ideas behind it."*

The book garnered significant acclaim in the United States, earning a national book award in 1937, and in Europe, where it was adapted into a movie in 1938 and inspired several television series. While some argue that Cronin himself never intended to advocate the formation of a national health program and was, in fact, opposed to state control, it is widely believed that the book influenced elections in 1945. This paved the way for NHS legislation under a labor-friendly government and underscored the pressing need for such a system.[8]

The NHS made the United Kingdom the first country to provide free medical care to all its citizens. Its establishment owes much to one physician's willingness to share his stories.

ONE FLEW OVER THE CUCKOO'S NEST

There is no more vivid portrayal of electroconvulsive therapy (ECT) than that depicted in the 1975 film "One Flew Over the Cuckoo's Nest." Jack Nicholson portrays the defiant R.P. McMurphy, who feigns insanity to escape a prison labor camp but ends up in a mental institution where he undergoes ECT as punishment for misbehavior rather than for mental illness.

The scene itself is harrowing. McMurphy is physically restrained by attendants as a mouthguard is forced into place. Without anesthesia, he endures the treatment with clenched teeth and shaking limbs. His face contorts in pain, and afterward, he is left gasping, groggy, and almost catatonic. The dramatic imagery terrified viewers and instilled fear in those who might face such treatment one day

The book version of the story, originally published in 1962, emerged during a period when many were challenging medical authority in what became known as the anti-psychiatry movement. This broad-based movement began in the 1960s and questions the legitimacy of psychiatric theory and practices. Despite ECT being a well-established and effective therapy by then, public support for such "barbaric" treatments waned. ECT usage declined in the 1960s and 1970s but saw a resurgence in the early 1980s, partly due to more positive accounts from writers like Norman Endler and Martha Manning.

Upending this discourse was renowned American physician and writer Sherwin Nuland, who practiced surgery for over three decades and taught at the Yale School of Medicine. Nuland authored numerous books based on his medical experiences, though lesser known was his personal battle with severe depression and mental illness in the 1970s. He spent significant time in psychiatric institutions and tried various medications before eventually considering ECT as a treatment.[9] When conventional treatments proved ineffective, his physicians suggested a pre-frontal lobotomy. Rather than opting for this drastic procedure, Nuland heeded a resident's advice and chose ECT instead.

His 2001 TED Talk, "How Electroshock Therapy Changed Me," reached millions of viewers and helped dispel misconceptions fostered by pop culture and the backlash of earlier decades. Nuland eloquently discusses the history and development of ECT, describing how it provided him with "relief, redemption, and second chances" in managing his severe depression.[10]

Today, ECT is administered to approximately 100,000 patients annually, with symptom improvement observed in 70%-90% of cases, sometimes after just one or two treatments. ECT is considered safe for pregnant women, teenagers, and the elderly, with no known long-term side effects, highlighting its safety and efficacy in contemporary medical practice.[11]

BEING MORTAL

End-of-life care in the United States is not only exorbitantly expensive but also often fails to meet the needs of patients. A recent study published in the *Journal of Pain and Symptom Management* revealed that the United

States ranks 43rd out of 81 countries in the quality of care provided to dying patients, with many expressing regrets over the treatments they receive.[12] This subpar care comes with a staggering price tag: Healthcare costs average $80,000 in the last 12 months of life, soaring to $150,000 over the last three years.[13] Shockingly, one quarter of all Medicare spending is allocated to care during the final year of life.[14]

Equally concerning is the lack of dignity and empathy within the U.S. medical system during this critical period. Chronic and debilitating illnesses often leave patients and their families feeling isolated. In hospitals, patients are stripped of their personal belongings and subjected to regimented routines, including intrusive procedures like frequent vital sign checks at all hours. Basic activities such as grooming, bathing, and feeding become arduous tasks requiring substantial assistance or full dependence on others. Many healthcare facilities have adopted sterile, impersonal environments that exacerbate the sense of isolation and discomfort.

Recognizing these shortcomings in end-of-life care, Atul Gawande, an American surgeon and author, interwove personal narratives from his own experiences and those of his patients and colleagues in his 2014 book *Being Mortal*:[15]

> *"Medicine has triumphed in modern times, transforming the dangers of childbirth, injury, and disease from harrowing to manageable. But when it comes to the inescapable realities of aging and death, what medicine can do often runs counter to what it should. Nursing homes, devoted above all to safety, battle with residents over the food they are allowed to eat and the choices they are allowed to make. Doctors, uncomfortable discussing patients' anxieties about death, fall back on false hopes and treatments that are actually shortening lives instead of improving them. And families go along with all of it."*

Among the myriad issues he discusses in the book, Gawande emphasizes that hospice care offers a more humane and cost-effective approach, potentially even extending life expectancy. While these concepts were well-established in medical circles, *Being Mortal* transcended academic settings and hospital corridors, resonating widely and even inspiring a popular PBS special of the same name. Since its publication in 2014,

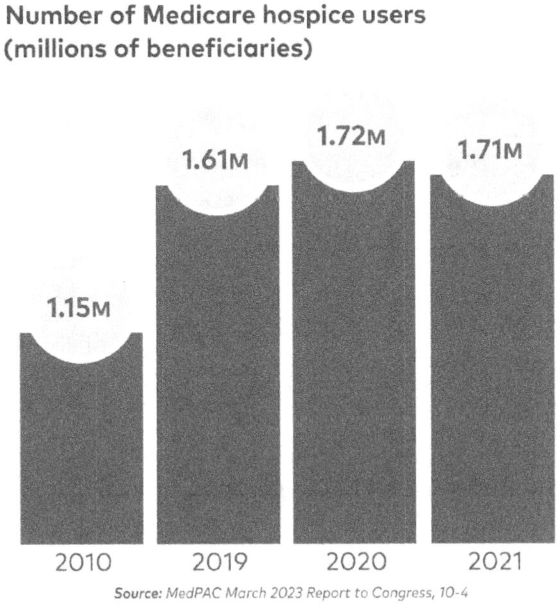

FIGURE 4. Number of Medicare Hospice Users. Source: Vick, R. (2023). *Innovations in End-of-Life Care.*[14]

hospice and palliative care have not only gained acceptance in end-of-life conversations but are increasingly seen as a superior model.

As illustrated in the Figure 4, Medicare-based hospice enrollment has surged by 30% since the release of *Being Mortal*. This increase can be attributed in part to a growing "death positive movement" and the emergence of services such as "death doulas," reflecting a broader societal shift towards prioritizing patient comfort over futile life extension efforts.[16]

Being Mortal, a collection of poignant stories from a surgeon's perspective on dignity and humanity within our healthcare system, has catalyzed these crucial discussions.

REBEL HEALTH

From 2000 to 2014, Susannah Fox served as associate director of the Internet Project at the Pew Research Center, where she led the health and technology portfolio. Pioneering participatory research methods, she explored the impact of information technology and social media on the healthcare industry, focusing particularly on individuals with chronic and rare conditions.

Transitioning to the role of chief technology officer at the U.S. Department of Health and Human Services (HHS) from 2015 to 2017, Fox fostered entrepreneurship and innovation overseeing 80,000 employees across 27 divisions. Her efforts aimed to leverage data and technology to enhance the nation's health and welfare.

In her 2024 book *Rebel Health: A Field Guide to the Patient-led Revolution in Medical Care,* Fox shares real-life patient narratives and chronicles the rise of the peer-to-peer health movement. This therapeutic method involves people who share a common experience or group membership to support each other in their health.

Throughout history, individuals grappling with illness and disability have sought solutions often absent in conventional healthcare. Whether through pre-internet support groups for rare diseases dating back to the 1970s or the contemporary hacking of diabetic medical technology, the public has connected to innovate their own remedies. Fox predicts that the next wave of healthcare innovation will emerge from the forefront of this patient-led revolution.

Fox's stories not only inspire those marginalized by the healthcare system but also provide a playbook for engaging patients and families in proactive health management and community well-being. She uses these narratives to encourage the medical community to evolve beyond the outdated paternal model of care. Collaborative partnerships between doctors and patients, Fox argues, yield better outcomes and pave the way for a more effective and inclusive healthcare approach in the 21st century.

IN MY HUMBLE OPINION

My journey into storytelling began in 2004 with my inaugural blog post on a blog entitled *In My Humble Opinion.* My mission was straightforward: to articulate the perspective from the other end of the stethoscope. Witnessing the gradual erosion of the doctor-patient relationship over time, I felt compelled to address the misconceptions perpetuated by various external influences. Back then, I lacked the comprehensive data and language that now shape this book, but the troubling transformation of this pivotal relationship was unmistakable.

Numerous factors, both constructive and detrimental, were reshaping doctors and patients into adversarial roles:

- The Institute of Medicine's report *To Err is Human*: Highlighting the prevalence and impact of medical errors, prompting reforms in healthcare quality and safety.
- Corporate America's efforts to commercialize medicine: Emphasizing profit motives and market-driven healthcare reforms, influencing healthcare delivery and patient outcomes.
- The evolving notion of work-life balance and increased expectations for fathers in child rearing: Shifting societal expectations on parental roles and its implications on healthcare professionals' well-being and patient care.
- The shift from the paternalistic model of patient care: Transitioning from hierarchical and authoritarian doctor-patient relationships to collaborative and patient-centered care models.
- The humanization of the American doctor: Recognizing the vulnerabilities, stresses, and burnout affecting healthcare professionals, leading to reforms in physician well-being and mental health support.
- The rise of the electronic medical record: Transformation of healthcare documentation and information management through digitalization, impacting healthcare efficiency, patient safety, and data accessibility.

What became abundantly clear was that doctors and patients were increasingly drifting apart, both physically and spiritually. This growing sense of disconnect from the American public left many physicians feeling more burned out than ever before. We found ourselves adrift in a vast sea of anger and disappointment.

The intimacy we once shared with our patients had eroded. As physicians, we had to acknowledge our role in this change. The practice of medicine was no longer reminiscent of the "good old days" our predecessors knew. We couldn't expect automatic respect based solely on our titles or positions. The world had evolved, and our patients sought more than just clinical expertise — they craved understanding and empathy. They yearned to converse with their doctors.

Patients were accustomed to a level of intimacy with their healthcare providers — sharing their most challenging stories and voicing their deepest fears. Meanwhile, doctors, no longer residing in their patients' neighborhoods or making house calls, inadvertently erected more barriers to intimacy than ever before. We had become disconnected from our patients' communities, social circles, and even their everyday rituals.

We had become isolated.

I sensed that the examination room was not the ideal setting to rebuild this intimacy. Patients entered with their own agendas, and there was still a place for objectivity and professional distance. To me, a public forum seemed far more fitting. What we desired wasn't intimacy with every individual patient, but rather a deeper and more profound connection with the entire community.

What better way to forge this connection than through our stories? Sharing our stories publicly, while respecting patient privacy, could serve as a lifeline to help our community see beyond the surface. How else could you understand a doctor's abrupt response or brief visit unless you knew that her thoughts were with a dying patient in the nearby hospital? Perhaps, as someone who might face a critical situation yourself one day, you would appreciate occasional distractions.

Stories dispel suspicion and clarify intentions. Intentions often speak louder than actions. Vulnerability forms the bridge between good intentions and imperfect actions. By sharing vulnerabilities, we cultivate intimacy. And through intimacy, we foster solidarity.

Stories are the bridge.

• • • • • •

My father passed away in the hospital while making rounds on his cancer patients. A small blood vessel in his brain ruptured, causing an intense headache followed by loss of consciousness and eventually a coma. His death wasn't attributed to workplace violence or trauma; it was a medical event that occurred while he happened to be in the hospital. It could have been a heart attack or a stroke.

Unlike my father, physicians often face injury or even death due to their jobs, a reality often overlooked by the media and the public at large.

According to the Bureau of Labor Statistics, healthcare workers experience more incidents of injury and illness compared to any other industry, including manufacturing and construction.[17] These injuries can include:[18]

- Sprains and strains.
- Slipped discs and other back injuries.
- Punctures and cuts.
- Broken bones.
- Head trauma.

Moreover, the World Health Organization (WHO) reports that 8%-38% of healthcare workers experience some form of physical violence during their careers.[19] A recent study of over 3,500 emergency medicine physicians revealed that 71% had witnessed assaults, with a staggering 47% having been physically assaulted themselves.[20]

Beyond accidental injuries and the risk of patient violence, there's another threat that is often too embarrassing and frightening to openly discuss: falling ill while caring for patients. This reality became painfully apparent during the COVID-19 pandemic, when many healthcare workers contracted the virus on the job.

In 2000, long before the era of COVID-19, there was another infection that instilled fear in many of us within the medical community. I myself worried that I might have contracted it at one point. For years, I kept this story hidden, afraid to share it even anonymously.

There's no fitting representation of what it feels like to go through medical school and especially residency. Samuel Shem's depiction in *The House of God* may be the closest. The mix of fear, exhaustion, wonder, and occasional joy is something that is not easily put into words. Yet, I also feel that many of my patients would say the same thing about what it feels like to be hospitalized or have a stay in the intensive care unit. Although medical training has been chosen and acute illness has not, I believe none of us are prepared for either, regardless whether we know it is coming.

While writing the piece "Stuck," I aimed to convey not only the lack of mercy and the challenges of medical training but also to impart an understanding of what it feels like to be a patient. Although non-physicians may not recognize it, behind the facade of every doctor is a person who has to confront their own mortality, sickness, and fear on a regular basis.

We share far more than sets us apart.

Stuck/Jordan Grumet

I have never told this story to anyone.

It was three a.m. and the call room was dark. The only light emanated from the small desk lamp on the nightstand. I sat on the bed and listened to the din of the hospital. It was finally quiet. The shades on the window were closed. As I looked down at the tourniquet, I knew this could change everything. My job, my health, my sanity. Such innocent objects: a needle, a syringe. I hesitated for about a second, and then I took the plunge. How did things get so complicated? I remembered back to one year ago.

The man lying on the bed was thin and appeared to be ill, as he curled into the fetal position. The doctor behind him gently pushed his head down into his legs. The patient contemplated his current position. He knew that he was dying. It had been years now and AIDS had ravaged his body. Somewhere in the depths of his soul he contemplated whether this was punishment for his excessive lifestyle, the drugs in particular. He had seen everyone he cared for either die or leave him.

As the doctor placed the spinal needle into the curvature of his back, the man thought about dignity. Something he hadn't felt in the last few years. It wasn't so much the pain of the spinal tap as it was the submission to someone else's will. Whether he had meningitis or not was no longer the point!

Suddenly the needle thrust inward and awakened him from his reverie. The pain shot through his body causing his back to jerk reflexively. He heard the doctor curse as the needle fell to the floor. The doctor excused himself and ran to the bathroom.

• • • • • •

As the patient jerked, I lost control of the needle. The force of his movement sent it bouncing into my finger and then to the floor.

"Shit!" I said loudly and ran to the bathroom.

I inspected the glove, which showed a small puncture wound. I tore it off and glared at my finger. No blood! Did I feel pain? I quickly turned the hot water on and vigorously scrubbed with soap. After five minutes my nerves calmed. It was three a.m. and I was tired and afraid.

I walked back into the patient's room, performed the lumbar puncture, and didn't tell a soul. And I did my best to never think about it again.

I submerged my fears. Little did I know they would come flying back in my face one year later.

• • • • • •

I was completely panicked. My wife had been sick for two weeks and I couldn't figure out why. She was having high fevers, weight loss, and horrible fatigue. The trip to the doctor that morning had been fruitless. The physical exam and blood tests were all normal. Yet the doctor couldn't explain why she had to rest twice just to make it up a flight of stairs. He assured us it was a virus and would likely pass.

With shock, my mind raced back to the night one year before. I thought about the needle stick and what that could have meant. I always figured that if I got sick it was one thing, but my wife? Of course the doctor hadn't performed an HIV test; there was no reason to suspect.

It was easy to find a label for the vial of blood. I quickly wrote an unintelligible scrawl in the place for the doctor's signature. I walked down the hall to the lab gingerly. I waited for the desk person to vacate so I could leave the sample in the drop box when no one would see me. Back in my call room I breathed a sigh of relief, cleaned up the wrappers, and the used needle and syringe. My fate, as well as that of my wife, would have to wait until morning.

• • • • • •

The attending walked confidently toward us the next day with a sneer on his face. As he strode into the nursing station, he addressed all of the residents at the same time.

"Which one of you dumbasses ordered an HIV test on Mr. Jones? Hardly a test that is indicated for an 85-year old with heart failure."

We all looked at him blankly for a minute and then I mustered enough confidence.

"So when should I start the cocktail?"

The attending smirked at my sarcasm, "Funny, Jordan! Of course it was negative!"

A week later my wife developed a sore throat and repeat blood testing showed she had infectious mononucleosis — mono. It would be 12 months before she felt normal again.

• • • • • •

The patient with AIDS died a few days after the botched lumbar puncture from complications of cryptococcal meningitis. He died alone; there was no next of kin or family to call. And I escaped unscathed (physically at least) with a promise to myself that I would never suffer alone with this again.

LIPSTICK ON A PIG

Paul and Matt were regular visitors to my office, arriving almost weekly with a trunk full of food and a backpack brimming with glossy materials and studies meticulously collated in a way that only a pharmaceutical representative could love. Matt would chat amicably with the front desk staff while Paul, without asking permission, would set up in our break room.

They quickly became the favored reps among our staff, earning themselves a cherished spot in our lunch rotation. I have to admit, I grew rather fond of them too. We engaged in spirited debates about the drugs they promoted and delved into discussions about the latest studies. They were eager to hear about my patients' experiences with their products and sought ways to better serve our community.

Over time, what started as a professional relationship morphed into a sort of friendship with me and the younger physicians in our office. They even sponsored a trip for all of us and our spouses to a champagne tasting downtown. They offered to compensate us for attending journal clubs and other activities where we discussed the value of the medicines they advocated. Although we were careful, I found myself regularly questioning whether I prescribed their medicines because they were truly the best choice, the most readily available in our sample closet, or simply because I liked Paul and Matt and enjoyed their company. These were significant ethical dilemmas.

A year passed filled with interactions, social events, and countless lunches. Paul and Matt became fixtures in our office, so familiar that some patients recognized them. What had initially seemed ethically dubious had become normalized through repetition. It was hard to see any harm in what we were doing, or so we convinced ourselves.

But I'll never forget the day a groundbreaking study published in a reputable journal revealed that one of Matt and Paul's main products was inferior to its competitors. When they visited us that day, they seemed more aggressive than usual, presenting study after study to sway us. Yet none of the physicians in our practice were convinced.

Science is science, and the data was unequivocal. It wasn't personal; Matt and Paul were good people, and some of us had even met their significant others. So, I was puzzled as they grew increasingly agitated. Their visits became tense, and the friendly lunches were replaced by company-paid speakers attempting to persuade us.

Eventually, Matt and Paul vanished. No more appreciative notes or trunks full of food. No more evenings out on the town celebrating their recent engagements. It turned out my assumption that we had transcended the typical sales rep-doctor relationship and become friends was fundamentally flawed.

To Matt and Paul, we were never friends. They may have treated us as such, but our interactions were ultimately transactional. Their goal was to sell more drugs, and we were their target. They had undergone extensive training provided by their company to cultivate relationships with their targets. In fact, I once took care of an actor who was paid handsomely to pose as a doctor and assist in training pharmaceutical reps on how to persuade skeptical physicians.

No matter what lipstick we put on the pig, I had been part of a year-long business transaction without even knowing it.

And so had all of us. We are all commodified, regardless of what pharmaceutical, insurance, or private equity companies may profess. They may claim to be our allies or genuinely interested in helping us. They may establish hotlines and participate in community events. But let us not forget: Doctors are not the only ones targeted. Profiting from patients is even more lucrative than from doctors.

When in doubt, follow the money. You'll discover that while the cost of our healthcare system skyrockets, the quality of care remains stagnant. Neither doctors nor patients benefit from this exorbitant spending spree. It is the third parties who profit.

THE REVOLUTION STARTS NOW

The only solution to our healthcare woes lies in revolution. We must upend the entrenched interests that have transformed patients from valued individuals into mere customers, monetized for the profit-driven agendas of corporations.

In Part One of this book, we explored the seismic shift that has reshaped the medical system over the past several decades. Patients, once held in high regard within society and our healthcare system, have now been reduced to mere customers. They have been capitalized, serving as fodder in the fiduciary responsibilities shared between businesses and their shareholders. Somehow, the core responsibilities enshrined in venerable documents like the Hippocratic oath have been forsaken.

This transformation began with the distortion of the doctor-patient relationship. Once a trusted cornerstone of our lives, physicians have been redefined as frenemies. Ostensibly, your doctor is present to provide assistance, yet various influences have portrayed physicians as a malevolent presence that generally does not prioritize society's best interests. Consequently, they have cast doubts on our competence through an artificially manufactured malpractice crisis and have falsely claimed that physicians' salaries are the root cause of our medical system's problems.

However, upon closer examination, the commodification of healthcare has primarily been orchestrated by various third parties poised to exploit both society's vulnerability regarding medical needs and the division between doctors and patients for their own gains.

Big Pharma is reducing their drug production while increasing prices, leveraging publicly funded research for profit. They not only circumvent federal regulations but also engage in aggressive public relations campaigns against any obstacles hindering their pursuit of greater profits. Meanwhile, they exploit the federal tax code to finance research and development, often outsourcing these activities to smaller, more efficient firms. Big Pharma's profit margins have reached unprecedented heights, enriching CEOs and boards with billions. Meanwhile, ordinary patients continue to pay exorbitant prices for medications that were more affordable in years past.

The misconduct of Big Pharma parallels that of big insurance companies. These insurers hinder our healthcare system with denials and lengthy prior authorizations for crucial medications and procedures. They engage in a strategic war of attrition, counting on many to give up rather than persist in fighting for their rightful care. Moreover, they neglect their duty to negotiate fair medical costs with hospitals and medical systems and show leniency toward obvious instances of fraud. Their motivation appears clear: The more they withhold in payouts, the more they retain in profits, simply passing on the costs through increased premiums. And in case you were worried, big insurance, like Big Pharma, is hauling in record profits and paying their executives a ludicrous sum of money. The equation is simple: Charge more and pay out less. Everyone wins, except, of course, the patients and caregivers.

Furthermore, not only have our patients been reduced to mere consumers, but there has also been a commodification of our healthcare systems. Hospitals, surgical centers, and medical practices, burdened by extensive governmental regulations, escalating technological demands, and fierce competition from corporate giants, are increasingly succumbing to acquisitions by private equity and venture capital firms.

These profit-driven entities often strip these healthcare systems of their infrastructure and assets in pursuit of quick financial gains. They willingly accept fines for regulatory breaches, calculating that non-compliance is cheaper than compliance. Their strategy is clear: Reduce operational costs, raise prices, and offload these businesses to other buyers before the full extent of the damage becomes apparent.

In Part Two, we explored how doctors themselves have been maneuvered into vulnerable positions. Politicians and corporate giants belittle them, focusing their attacks on competence (malpractice), access (time), and incentives (money). Their aim is to erode trust between doctors and patients, dividing us to distract from the draining of our financial resources.

The Institute of Medicine's report *To Err is Human* drives this assault. It paints a distorted picture suggesting that a significant majority of hospital patients succumb due to medical errors. This misrepresentation relies on flawed data and exaggerated extrapolations, creating a grim portrayal of healthcare plagued by mistakes and misconduct. Exploiting this misinformation, lawyers spur communities to flood the courts with medical malpractice claims. The reality, however, is starkly different. The majority of malpractice claims are dismissed before reaching trial, and a substantial number of those that do proceed find no evidence of malpractice. Despite this, patients and their families endure prolonged, often harrowing legal battles, while physicians face grueling public scrutiny that can lead to PTSD. Ultimately, the primary beneficiaries are the lawyers.

Compounding this issue, extensive data illustrate the exorbitant costs of our litigious culture. Billions of dollars are squandered on defensive medicine aimed at mitigating legal risks, driving up malpractice premiums to unsustainable levels. We bear the brunt of these escalating costs.

The growing physical and emotional gap between doctors and patients is exacerbated by mounting governmental regulations and the cumbersome burden of electronic medical records. Studies indicate that primary care physicians would require more than 24 hours a day to adhere to all current guidelines for a single day's caseload.

Consequently, physicians are experiencing unprecedented levels of burnout, a condition marked not only by physical exhaustion but also profound moral injury. Many are leaving clinical practice altogether, pursuing non-clinical careers, or tragically, even taking their own lives at alarming rates.

Something has to change.

Moreover, it seems that the government is increasingly at odds with physicians. Laws ostensibly designed to safeguard society, such as the Affordable Care Act's creation of ACOs, the False Claims Act, anti-kickback and Stark laws, alongside numerous state statutes, are not only complicating physicians' lives but also imposing excessive penalties for often unintentional mistakes.

Rather than focusing on penalizing deliberate wrongdoers, these laws are transforming most physicians into unintentional offenders. Both the virtuous and the culpable are bearing the consequences.

In Part Three, having painted such a bleak picture, I shift focus to proposing solutions to the challenges we face. The only viable remedy is revolution. Incremental steps are insufficient against the entrenched power and influence of these third parties obstructing our progress.

Revolutionary change can only materialize when the principal stakeholders in a failing system unite with a single voice. In today's healthcare landscape, the primary stakeholders are clear: the patients who depend on care, and the doctors (alongside other caregivers) who deliver it. Period.

Yet, we are not only divided by these third parties; we face an even more formidable challenge — an intimacy gap. Patients enter the exam room and share their deepest secrets, worries, and fears. Meanwhile, doctors often remain detached, maintaining a paternalistic facade of objectivity. Naturally, patients don't feel connected to us; we impart medical knowledge without revealing who we are. To bridge this gap, we must cultivate intimacy to forge alliances.

Breaking through this barrier requires us to share our stories — not confined to the exam room but broadcast to the world. By revealing our hearts, sacrifices, and regrets, we allow others to see themselves in our triumphs and failures. I am not just the doctor who attends to your father in his final moments, but also the decision-maker haunted by guilt for not alleviating his suffering. I am the grieving friend losing someone I've known for years. I am not immune to life's struggles; I stand alongside you in the arena — we are allies in this battle.

When doctors and patients unite through shared storytelling, revolutions can manifest on both grand and modest scales. For instance, in the United Kingdom, this collaboration helped pave the way for universal healthcare. Similarly, in the United States, it brought about critical reforms in industries like meatpacking, prioritizing food safety and protecting workers.

Smaller revolutions are also frequent when doctors recount their experiences. Atul Gawande's exploration of dignity in end-of-life care or Sherwin Nuland's TED Talk on the transformative power of electroconvulsive therapy are prime examples. These narratives not only enlighten but also inspire change.

If we are earnest about fostering change, we must amplify our storytelling efforts — creating more expansive, more impactful stories that resonate deeply and bring about action.

IMAGINE IF YOU CAN

Regina Holliday's beloved husband, Fred, tragically passed away in the hospital on June 19, 2009, at the age of 39. Overwhelmed with grief and frustrated by the difficult access to his medical records, Holliday did not seek out malpractice lawyers. Instead, she turned her attention to a gas station wall several miles from the U.S. Capitol and the White House. There, she created her mural titled "73 Cents," depicting the harrowing experience of Fred's hospital transfer and the shocking news that she would have to pay 73 cents per page and wait up to 21 days to obtain his medical records, despite the information being readily available for printing from a computer screen. She feared Fred didn't have 21 days left.

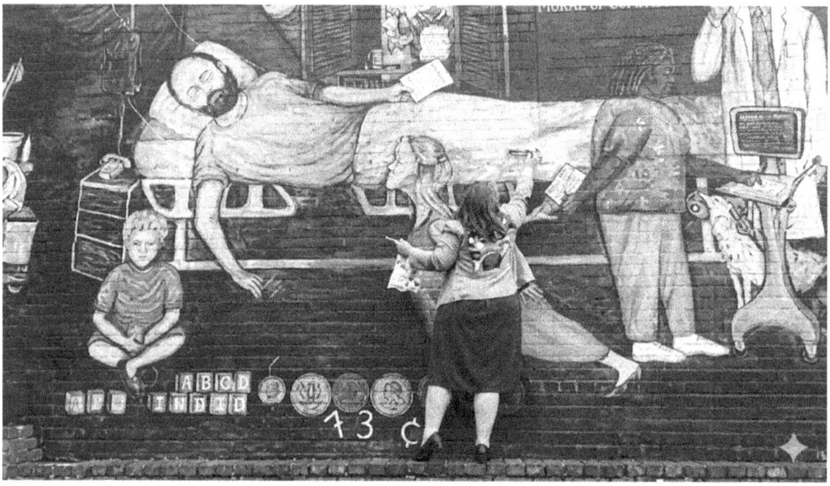

After attending her first medical conference in 2009, Holliday was struck by the stark absence of patient representation among those in positions of power, who were typically adorned in business suits. In response, she decided to paint a series of artworks on the back of blazers worn by health advocates, including doctors, at scientific meetings.

Over a decade later, the Walking Gallery has grown to include 466 members, each proudly displaying patient stories painted on their backs. They attend medical conferences where patient speakers are often notably absent from both the podium and the audience. The Walking Gallery now spans six continents, symbolizing a global movement for patient advocacy and awareness within healthcare settings.

One of those walkers is Dave Debronkart, widely recognized as e-Patient Dave, whose journey surviving kidney cancer has propelled him into activism for healthcare transformation, particularly advocating for participatory medicine and personal health data rights.

Debronkart partnered with his personal physician, renowned Harvard primary care doctor Danny Sands, to co-found The Society for Participatory Medicine. This organization champions a movement where patients and healthcare professionals collaborate actively, encouraging one another and sharing their stories.

Another co-founder and fellow Walking Gallery member, Susannah Fox, previously served as associate director of the Pew Research Center's Internet and American Life Project, where she illuminated healthcare narratives through data. In 2015, she assumed the role of chief technology officer at the U.S. Department of Health & Human Services, a position she held until 2017.

Our stories fuel our world!

Imagine, if you can, a future where we hold the reins to our own narratives. Where we wield the power. Where more family members like Regina Holliday can express their stories through art and murals rather than relying on the tired half-truths of the American medicolegal complex. Picture a world where the tales of more e-patients, such as Dave Debronkart, overshadow the inflated claims perpetuated by medical records companies more concerned with profits than user experience. Envision doctors like Danny Sands sharing their insights, and patient advocates and government officials like Susannah Fox attending regulatory meetings adorned with a patient's story on their backs.

In this future, a hypothetical account detailing the injustices of our medical system, experienced firsthand by a single doctor in the field could one day lead to Medicare for all. Similar to Dr. A.J. Cronin's groundbreaking book *The Citadel,* which influenced the creation of the National Health Service in the United Kingdom.

These are our stories. This is our humanity. If we want to cleave the bonds of third-party leverage that hold us back and bankrupts our system, we have to tell them.

We have to tell them.

Glossary

Accountable care organizations (ACOs) are groups of healthcare providers that work together to improve the quality of care for a specific group.

American Medical Association is an association whose purpose is "to promote the science and art of medicine and the betterment of public health."

The antipsychiatry movement is a broad-based movement that began in the 1960s and questions the legitimacy of psychiatric theory and practices.

Carvedilol is a common blood pressure medicine from the beta-blocker family.

A contingency agreement is a fee arrangement in which an attorney or firm agrees that the payment of legal fees will be based upon the successful outcome of the case.

Corporate practice of medicine doctrine prohibits corporations from practicing medicine or employing a physician to provide professional medical services.

Defensive medicine is the practice of ordering unnecessary tests to reduce the risk of malpractice litigation.

Disease mongering is a negative term for the practice of expanding the diagnostic boundaries of illnesses and raising public awareness of them to increase treatment markets.

EHR is an electronic health record.

EMR is an electronic medical record.

End-of-life secretions, also known as terminal respiratory secretions (RTS) or "death rattle," are a natural part of the dying process for many people who are terminally ill.

False Claims Act (FCA) provides that any person who knowingly submits, or causes to submit, false claims to the government is liable for three times the government's damages plus a penalty that is linked to inflation.

Food and Drug Administration (FDA) protects the public health by assuring the safety, efficacy, and security of biological products and medical devices.

Gag laws are laws that restrict physicians from asking their patients specific questions.

HIPAA stands for Health Insurance Portability and Accountability Act, a federal law passed in 1996 to protect medical records and personal health information.

Hippocratic Oath is an oath stating the obligations and proper conduct of doctors, formally taken by those beginning medical practice.

Information blocking is intentionally interfering with the flow of information between different EHR systems.

Interoperability is the ability of different health data systems to share and use data securely, regardless of location, to improve patient care and community health.

Key opinion leader (KOL) is a trusted, influential professional with expertise in a particular field or industry who can sway public opinion about products, services, or matters.

Maslach Burnout Inventory (MBI), the leading measure of burnout, is validated by the extensive research conducted for more than 35 years.

Meaningful use is a program run by the Centers for Medicare & Medicaid Services (CMS) that encourages healthcare providers to use electronic health records (EHR) technology in ways that benefit patients and providers.

Medical downcoding is a billing practice in which a procedure or service is billed at a lower level than what was actually provided.

Medical upcoding is a type of healthcare fraud that occurs when a provider submits inaccurate billing codes to an insurance company for a medical procedure or treatment to increase reimbursement.

MMSS stands for medical malpractice stress syndrome which refers to the traumatic experience of being sued for malpractice.

Moral injury (MI) is a distressing psychological, behavioral, social, and sometimes spiritual response to an event that violates or betrays an individual's moral values or beliefs.

Narrative exposure therapy (NET) is a treatment approach for trauma disorders like PTSD where sufferers create a chronological narrative of traumatic life events.

Narrative medicine is medicine practiced with narrative competence to recognize, absorb, interpret, and be moved by the stories of illness.

Patent foramen ovale (PFO) is a hole between the left and right atria (upper chambers) of the heart. This hole exists in everyone before birth, but most often closes shortly after birth.

Peer-to-peer health movement is a therapeutic method that involves people who share a common experience or group membership to support each other in their health.

Plaintiff is a person who brings a case against another person in a court of law.

Posttraumatic stress disorder (PTSD) is a psychiatric disorder that may occur in people who have experienced or witnessed a traumatic event.

Prior authorization is a requirement from a health insurance company that a doctor obtains approval before using a medicine.

Private equity (PE) is a type of investment that involves buying and managing companies that are not publicly traded or listed on a stock exchange.

Professional distance in medicine, also known as professional boundaries, is the distance a healthcare professional should maintain with their patient to ensure quality care.

Retroactive denial is the reversal of a previously paid claim, where you become responsible for payment.

Safe harbor exception in the federal anti-kickback statute is a set of regulations that defines payment practices that are not considered offenses under the law.

Standard of care is what a reasonable physician would do in identical circumstances.

Summons is an order to appear before a judge.

Three-Minute Mental Makeover (3MMM) is an uncomplicated but research-backed journaling technique that may significantly reduce stress with lasting effects.

To Err is Human: Building a Safer Health System is a 1999 report by the Institute of Medicine (IOM) Committee that called for a national effort to reduce preventable medical errors in the United States.

Universal basic coverage (UBC) is a proposal for a health insurance system that provides access to essential healthcare regardless of resources.

Walking Gallery is an advocacy movement and artist-led project that aims to start conversations about healthcare by painting patient stories on people's jackets.

Some Contemporary Physician Writers and a Few of Their Notable Titles

Atul Gawande, MD, MPH, holds the John and Cyndy Fish Chair in Surgery at Brigham and Women's Hospital and is the Samuel O. Thier Professor of the Practice of Surgery at Harvard Medical School. He is the former assistant administrator for global health at the U.S. Agency for International Development, where he oversaw a bureau that managed more than $4 billion with a footprint of more than 900 staff committed to advancing equitable delivery of public health approaches around the world. He is the author of:

- *Being Mortal: Medicine and What Matters in the End*
- *The Checklist Manifesto: How to Get Things Right*
- *Complications: A Surgeon's Notes on an Imperfect Science*

Abraham Verghese, MD, MACP, is an American physician and professor of the theory and practice of medicine and vice chair of education at Stanford University Medical School. He is the author of:

- *Cutting for Stone*
- *My Own Country: A Doctor's Story*
- *The Tennis Partner: A Doctor's Story of Friendship and Loss*

Siddhartha Mukherjee, MD, is a physician, researcher, and associate professor of medicine at Columbia University, and an oncologist at the university's medical center. He is the author of:

- *The Emperor of All Maladies: A Biography of Cancer*
- *The Gene: An Intimate History*

Oliver Sacks, MD, was a British neurologist who won acclaim for his sympathetic case histories of patients with unusual neurological disorders.

- *The Man Who Mistook His Wife for a Hat*
- *Awakenings*
- *An Anthropologist on Mars*

Paul Kalanithi, MD, was a neurosurgeon who graduated cum laude from the Yale School of Medicine. He completed his residency training in neurological surgery and a postdoctoral fellowship in neuroscience at Stanford, during which he received the American Academy of Neurological Surgery's highest award for research. He died in March 2015 from metastatic lung cancer at the age of 37.

- *When Breath Becomes Air*

Michael Crichton was an American writer known for his thoroughly researched popular thrillers, which often deal with the potential ramifications of advancing technology. He studied at Harvard Medical School but never practiced medicine. He created the hit TV series *ER*. His books include:

- *The Andromeda Strain*
- *Jurassic Park*

Jerome Groopman, MD, holds the Dina and Raphael Recanati Chair of Medicine at Harvard Medical School and is chief of experimental medicine at Beth Israel Deaconess Medical Center in Boston. He has published more than 150 scientific articles. He is also and is a staff writer at The New Yorker. His books include:

- *How Doctors Think*
- *The Anatomy of Hope: How People Prevail in the Face of Illness*
- *Your Medical Mind*

Danielle Ofri, MD, is an attending physician at Bellevue Hospital and clinical professor of medicine at New York University School of Medicine. Books include:

- *When We Do Harm*
- *What Patients Say, What Doctors Hear*
- *What Doctors Feel*
- *Singular Intimacies: Becoming a Doctor at Bellevue*

Gavin Francis is a Scottish physician and a writer on travel and medical matters. He was raised in Fife, Scotland and now is a GP in Edinburgh. His books include:

- Adventures in Human Being

- *Intensive Care: A GP, a Community, and COVID-19*
- *The Unfragile Mind: Making Sense of Mental Health*

Sherwin B. Nuland, MD, FACS, was a practicing surgeon for 30 years and treated more than 10,000 patients — then became a writer and speaker on topics of life and death, our minds, our morality, aging and the human spirit.

- *Doctors: The Biography of Medicine*
- *How We Die: Reflections on Life's Final Chapter*

Richard Selzer was a surgeon who completed a surgical internship and residency at Yale University and remained as assistant clinical professor of surgery until 1985 in addition to maintaining a private practice. His books include:

- *Mortal Lessons: Notes on the Art of Surgery*
- *Confessions of a Knife*

Richard Preston is a bestselling author and writer for *The New Yorker* who has written books about infectious disease, bioterrorism, and other subjects. His books include:

- *The Hot Zone: The Terrifying True Story of the Origins of the Ebola Virus*
- *Cannibals, Killer Viruses, and Other Journeys to the Edge of Science*

Perri Klass, MD, is an American pediatrician who has published extensively about her medical training and pediatric practice. Among her subjects have been the issues of women in medicine, relationships between doctors and patients, and children and literacy. Books include:

- *Treatment Kind and Fair: Letters to a Young Doctor*
- *Baby Doctor: A Pediatrician's Training*

David Agus, MD, is one of the world's leading doctors and pioneering biomedical researchers. He is the founding director and co-CEO of the Ellison Institute of Technology and a professor of medicine and engineering at the University of Southern California. Books include:

- *The End of Illness*
- *A Short Guide to a Long Life*
- *The Lucky Years*

Pauline Chen, MD, is a surgeon who has been the recipient of numerous awards including the UCLA Outstanding Physician of the Year Award in 1999 and the George Longstreth Humanness Award at Yale for most exemplifying empathy, kindness, and care in an age of advancing technology. Publications include:

- Final Exam: A Surgeon's Reflections on Mortality
- *Doctor and Patient* blog

Victoria Sweet, MD, is an American physician and advocate for what is termed "slow medicine." She is also a historian of medicine who has studied the writings of Hildegard of Bingen, a 12th century German abbess and medical therapist. Books include:

- *God's Hotel: A Doctor, a Hospital, and a Pilgrimage to the Heart of Medicine*
- *Slow Medicine: The Way to Healing*

Mukesh Kapila, MD, is emeritus professor of global health and humanitarian affairs at the University of Manchester, UK. Books include:

- *Against a Tide of Evil: How One Man Became the Whistleblower to the First Mass Murder of the Twenty-First Century*
- *No Stranger to Kindness*

Kay Redfield Jamison is the Dalio Professor in Mood Disorders, professor of psychiatry at the Johns Hopkins University School of Medicine, and co-director of the Johns Hopkins Mood Disorders Center. She is also honorary professor of English at the University of St. Andrews in Scotland. Books include:

- *An Unquiet Mind: A Memoir of Moods and Madness*
- *Touched with Fire*
- *Fires in the Dark: Healing the Unquiet Mind*

References

Introduction

1. Mary Lou Retton's Net Worth. https://parade.com/celebrities/mary-lou-retton-net-worth.
2. Norris L. 6 lessons Mary Lou Retton's health scare can teach us about coverage. HealthInsurance.org blog. January 23, 2024. Accessed April 3, 2026. https://www.healthinsurance.org/blog/6-lessons-mary-lou-rettons-health-scare-can-teach-us-about-coverage/#:~:text=On%20the%20Today%20Show%2C%20Retton,going%20to%20happen%20to%20me%3F%E2%80%9D.
3. Kliff S. Mary Lou Retton crowdfunded her medical debt, like many thousands of others. *New York Times*. October 12, 2023. Accessed April 3, 2026. https://www.nytimes.com/2023/10/12/health/mary-lou-retton-medical-bills-crowdfunding.html
4. Big pharma is running out the clock on American patients. AHIP. Accessed January 3, 2023. https://www.ahip.org/reject-big-pharmas-drug-pricing-distractions-protect-your-bargaining-power.
5. Singh Y, Radhakrishnan N, Adler L, Whaley C. Growth of private equity and hospital consolidation in primary care and price implications. *JAMA Health Forum*. 2025;6(1):e244935. doi:10.1001/jamahealthforum.2024.4935.
6. Zhu JM, Song Z. The growth of private equity in US health care: impact and outlook. NIHCM Foundation. National Institute for Health Care Management. Accessed February 1, 2023. https://nihcm.org/publications/the-growth-of-private-equity-in-us-health-care-impact-and-outlook.
7. Institute of Medicine (US) Committee on Quality of Health Care in America, Kohn LT, Corrigan JM, Donalddson MS (eds). *To Err Is Human: Building a Safer Health System*. Washington, DC: National Academies Press;1999. https://doi.org/10.17226/9728.

Part One: When Patients Become Customers

1. The Legacy of Henrietta Lacks. Johns Hopkins Medicine. Accessed January 6, 2024. https://www.hopkinsmedicine.org/henrietta-lacks.
2. PBS NewsHour. Family of Henrietta Lacks, whose cells were taken for medical advancement, settles with company that profited. PBS. August 21, 2023. Accessed January 6, 2024. https://www.pbs.org/newshour/nation/family-of-henrietta-lacks-whose-cells-were-taken-for-medical-advancement-settles-with-company-that-profited.
3. Henrietta Lacks' estate sues Thermo Fisher. CBS News. October 4, 2021. Accessed January 12, 2023. https://www.cbsnews.com/news/henrietta-lacks-cells-estate-sues-thermo-fisher/.

4. The history of healthcare in America: from the 1700s to now. JP Griffin Group. Accessed January 7, 2024. https://cdn2.hubspot.net/hubfs/457237/JP_Griffin_Group_The_History_of_Healthcare_in_America.pdf.
5. Carroll A. The real reason the U.S. has employer-sponsored health insurance. *The New York Times*. September 2017. Accessed January 7, 2024. https://www.nytimes.com/2017/09/05/upshot/the-real-reason-the-us-has-employer-sponsored-health-insurance.html.
6. A history of the pharmaceutical industry. Pharmaphorum. September 1, 2020. Accessed January 7, 2024. https://pharmaphorum.com/r-d/a_history_of_the_pharmaceutical_industry.

Chapter One: Is Your Doctor Your Frenemy? (The Patient's View)

1. Johnson B. Letter to the editor. *The Los Angeles Times*. May 23, 2021. Accessed January 7, 2024. https://www.latimes.com/opinion/story/2021-05-23/blaming-doctors-america-has-no-healthcare-system.
2. Allen M. Why your health insurer doesn't care about your big bills. *ProPublica*. Accessed January 8, 2024. https://www.propublica.org/article/why-your-health-insurer-does-not-care-about-your-big-bills.
3. Hospital prices. August 22, 2021. *The New York Times*. Accessed January 8, 2024. https://www.nytimes.com/interactive/2021/08/22/upshot/hospital-prices.html.
4. Kane CK. Recent changes in physician practice arrangements: private practice dropped to less than 50 percent of physicians in 2020. *AMA Policy Research Perspectives*. May 2021. Accessed January 8, 2024. https://www.ama-assn.org/system/files/2021-05/2020-prp-physician-practice-arrangements.pdf.
5. Ornstein C, Weber T, Jones RG. We found over 700 doctors who were paid more than a million dollars by drug and medical device companies. *ProPublica*. October 17, 2019. Accessed January 8, 2024. https://www.propublica.org/article/we-found-over-700-doctors-who-were-paid-more-than-a-million-dollars-by-drug-and-medical-device-companies.
6. Kshirsagar R, Vu P. The pharmaceutical industry's role in U.S. medical education. In-Training. April 3, 2016. Accessed January 10, 2024. https://in-training.org/drugged-greed-pharmaceutical-industrys-role-us-medical-education-10639.
7. Pham-Kanter G, Mello MM, Lehmann LS, Campbell EG, Carpenter D. Public awareness of and contact with physicians who receive industry payments: a national survey. *J Gen Intern Med*. 2017;32:767–774. Accessed January 10, 2024. https://doi.org/10.1007/s11606-017-4012-3.
8. Baker D. The problem of doctors' salaries. *Politico*. October 25, 2017. Accessed January 10, 2024. https://www.politico.com/agenda/story/2017/10/25/doctors-salaries-pay-disparities-000557/.

9. McKenna J. Medscape physician compensation report 2024: bigger checks, yet doctors still see an underpaid profession. Medscape. April 12, 2024. Accessed May 10, 2024. https://www.medscape.com/slideshow/2024-compensation-overview-6017073#2.
10. AMA to fund graduate medical education, address physician shortages. AMA Press Release. June 12, 2019. Accessed January 10, 2024. https://www.ama-assn.org/press-center/press-releases/ama-fund-graduate-medical-education-address-physician-shortages#:~:text=These%20include%20the%20Resident%20Physician,affecting%20hospitals%20that%20host%20small.
11. Jubbal K. America's doctor shortage explained. Med School Insiders. July 16, 2022. Accessed January 12, 2024. https://medschoolinsiders.com/pre-med/americas-doctor-shortage-explained/.
12. AUAMED. Medical school tuition in USA and Canada: 2024 comparison. American University of Antigua blog. March 30, 2024. Accessed April 3, 2026. https://www.auamed.org/blog/how-much-is-medical-school-in-canada/#:~:text=On%20average%2C%20Canadian%20citizens%20and,fee%20of%20%2427%2C304%20per%20year.
13. *2022 physician compensation report*. Medscape. 2022. Accessed January 12, 2024. https://www.medscape.com/sites/public/physician-comp/2022.
14. Dyrda L. Physician vs. healthcare CEO pay: 5 notes. *Becker's ASC Review*. January 3, 2022. Accessed January 12, 2024. https://www.beckersasc.com/asc-news/physician-vs-healthcare-ceo-pay-5-notes.html#:~:text=By%20comparison%2C%20healthcare%20CEO%20total,%2C%20CEO%20of%20Nashville%2C%20Tenn.
15. Du JY, Rascoe AS, Marcus RE. The growing executive-physician wage gap in major US nonprofit hospitals and burden of nonclinical workers on the US healthcare system. *Clin Orthop Relat Res*. 2018; 476(10):1910-1919. https://doi.org/10.1097/CORR.0000000000000394.
16. Majority Staff Report for the U.S. Senate Committee on Health, Education, Labor, and Pensions. The Pharma Pandemic Profiteers. February 15, 2023. https://www.sanders.senate.gov/wp-content/uploads/Pharma-Exec-Compensation-Report.pdf.
17. Herman B. Seven health insurance CEOs raked in a record $283 million last year. STAT News. May 12, 2022. Accessed January 14, 2024. https://www.statnews.com/2022/05/12/health-insurance-ceos-raked-in-record-pay-during-covid/.
18. Kononchuk E. Average software developer salaries: rate comparison by country. Qubit Labs. March 4, 2026. Accessed April 3, 2026. https://qubit-labs.com/average-software-developer-salaries-salary-comparison-country/.

19. Galan S. Average annual CEO compensation worldwide. Statista. November 28, 2025. Accessed April 3, 2026. https://www.statista.com/statistics/424154/average-annual-ceo-compensation-worldwide/.
20. Reinhardt UE. The role of prices in health care spending. *The New York Times.* September 16, 2011. Accessed January 14, 2024. https://archive.nytimes.com/economix.blogs.nytimes.com/2011/09/16/the-role-of-prices-in-health-care-spending/?ref=health.
21. Henry TA. Medicine's great resignation: 1 in 5 doctors plan to exit in 2 years. American Medical Association. January 18, 2022. Accessed January 18, 2024. https://www.ama-assn.org/practice-management/physician-health/medicine-s-great-resignation-1-5-doctors-plan-exit-2-years#:~:text=One%20in%20five%20physicians%20say,to%20recently%20published%20survey%20research.
22. Trust in doctors has plummeted by 5%. What can be done? Advisory Board. Posted February 16, 2018. Updated March 24, 2023. Accessed January 18, 2024. https://www.advisory.com/daily-briefing/2018/02/16/trusting-medical-professionals.
23. Birkhauer J, Gaab J, Kossowsky J, Hasler S, Krummenacher P, *et al.* Trust in the health care profession and health outcome: a meta-analysis. *PloS One.* 2017;12(20:e0170988. https://doi.org/10.1371/journal.pone.0170988.
24. NORC at the University of Chicago. Surveys of trust in the U.S. health care system. May 21, 2021. Accessed April 3, 2026. https://www.norc.org/PDFs/ABIM%20Foundation/20210520_NORC_ABIM_Foundation_Trust%20in%20Healthcare_Part%201.pdf.
25. Wikipedia Contributors. *Edward Rosenbaum.* Wikipedia. Latest revision March 24, 2026. Accessed October 9, 2024. https://en.wikipedia.org/wiki/Edward_Rosenbaum.
26. Institute of Medicine (US) Committee on Quality of Health Care in America, Kohn LT, Corrigan JM, Donaldson MS, (eds.). *To Err Is Human: Building a Safer Health System.* Washington, DC: National Academy Press; 2000. https://doi.org/10.17226/9728.
27. What is patient-centered care? *NEJM Catalyst.* January 1, 2017. Accessed October 10, 2024. https://catalyst.nejm.org/doi/full/10.1056/CAT.17.0559.

Chapter Two: Does a Spoonful of Sugar Really Help the Medicine Go Down?

1. FDA orders halt to marketing of unapproved single-ingredient oral colchicine. Fierce Pharma. October 1, 2010. Accessed January 21, 2024. https://www.fiercepharma.com/pharma/fda-orders-halt-to-marketing-of-unapproved-single-ingredient-oral-colchicine.

2. Staton T. Takeda snaps up URL Pharma in $800M+ deal. Fierce Pharma. April 11, 2012. Accessed January 20, 2024. https://www.fiercepharma.com/m-a/takeda-snaps-up-url-pharma-800m-deal#:~:text=Takeda%20Pharmaceutical%20(%24TKPHF.PK,million%20for%20URL%20last%20year.
3. The budget and economic outlook: 2021 to 2031. Congressional Budget Office. February 2021. Accessed January 20, 2024. https://www.cbo.gov/publication/56970.
4. Frank RG, Hannick K. Five things to understand about pharmaceutical R&D. Brookings Institute blog. June 2, 2022. Accessed January 20, 2024. https://www.brookings.edu/blog/usc-brookings-schaeffer-on-health-policy/2022/06/02/five-things-to-understand-about-pharmaceutical-rd/.
5. Dranove D, Garthwaite C, Hermosilla M. The impact of pharmaceutical innovation on public health. National Bureau of Economic Research Working Paper. June 2014. Accessed January 20, 2024. https://www.nber.org/system/files/working_papers/w20212/w20212.pdf.
6. Mazzucato M. Op-Ed: How taxpayers prop up Big Pharma and how to cap that. *The Los Angeles Times.* October 27, 2015. Accessed January 21, 2024. https://www.latimes.com/opinion/op-ed/la-oe-1027-mazzucato-big-pharma-prices-20151027-story.html.
7. Cleary EG, Beierlein JM, Khanuja NS, Ledley FD, McNamee LN. Contribution of NIH funding to new drug approvals 2010-2016. *Proc Natl Acad Sci USA.* 2018;115(10):2329–2334. Accessed January 21, 2024. https://doi.org/10.1073/pnas.1715368115.
8. Bulik BS. Never say die: senators take another stab at repealing pharma DTC tax write-off. Fierce Pharma. March 2, 2018. Accessed January 21, 2024. https://www.fiercepharma.com/marketing/never-say-die-senators-taking-another-stab-at-repealing-pharma-dtc-ad-tax.
9. Komendant E. Pharmaceutical patent abuse: to infinity and beyond. Association for Accessible Medicines blog. Accessed January 21, 2024. https://accessiblemeds.org/resources/blog/pharmaceutical-patent-abuse-infinity-and-beyond#:~:text=In%20a%20recent%20report%20from,arthritis%20and%20other%20chronic%20conditions.
10. Fox E. How pharma companies game the system to keep drugs expensive. *Harvard Business Review.* April 6, 2017. Accessed January 21, 2024. https://hbr.org/2017/04/how-pharma-companies-game-the-system-to-keep-drugs-expensive.
11. Bakkila BF, Basu S, Lipska KJ. Catastrophic spending on insulin in the United States, 2017–18. *Health Aff (Millwood).* 2022;41(7):1053-1060. https://doi.org/10.1377/hlthaff.2021.01788.

12. Fernandez G. Why Eli Lilly's insulin price cap announcement matters. Johns Hopkins Bloomberg School of Public Health. Published March 13, 2023. Updated March 15, 2023. Accessed January 23, 2024. https://publichealth.jhu.edu/2023/eli-lilly-lowers-insulin-prices#:~:text=The%20burden%20is%20even%20greater,available%20income%20on%20the%20drug.
13. Lovelace B. Why is insulin still so expensive for diabetes patients in the US? NBC News. July 24, 2022. Accessed January 23, 2024. https://www.nbcnews.com/health/health-news/why-insulin-so-expensive-diabetes-united-states-rcna39295.
14. White House fact sheet: President Biden's cap on the cost of insulin could benefit millions of Americans in all 50 states. March 2, 2023. Accessed January 23, 2024. https://bidenwhitehouse.archives.gov/briefing-room/statements-releases/2023/03/02/fact-sheet-president-bidens-cap-on-the-cost-of-insulin-could-benefit-millions-of-americans-in-all-50-states/.
15. Kansteiner F. Lilly slashes insulin prices by 70%, caps out-of-pocket costs at $35 in major access overhaul. Fierce Pharma. March 1, 2023. Accessed April 3, 2026. https://www.fiercepharma.com/pharma/lilly-slashes-insulin-prices-70-caps-out-pocket-costs-35-major-access-overhaul.
16. Justice Department announces global resolution of criminal and civil investigations with opioid manufacturer Purdue Pharma and civil settlement with members of the Sackler family. U.S. Department of Justice Office of Public Affairs Press Release. October 21, 2020. Accessed January 24, 2024. https://www.justice.gov/opa/pr/justice-department-announces-global-resolution-criminal-and-civil-investigations-opioid.
17. Mann B, Bebinger M. Purdue Pharma, Sacklers reach $6 billion deal with state attorneys general. NPR. March 3, 2022. Accessed January 24, 2024. https://www.npr.org/2022/03/03/1084163626/purdue-sacklers-oxycontin-settlement#:~:text=Court%20filings%20show%20the%20family,brought%20a%20growing%20public%20backlash.
18. Cooper R. Disease mongering. Wiley Online Library. June 15, 2020. Accessed January 24, 2024. https://onlinelibrary.wiley.com/doi/10.1002/9781444367072.wbiee039.pub2.
19. Moynihan R, Heath I, Henry D. Selling sickness: the pharmaceutical industry and disease mongering. *BMJ*. 2002 Apr 13;324(7342):886-91. https://doi.org/10.1136/bmj.324.7342.886.
20. Ryan H, Girion L, Glover S. OxyContin goes global—'we're only just getting started.' *The Los Angeles Times*. December 18, 2016. Accessed January 24, 2023. https://www.latimes.com/projects/la-me-oxycontin-part3/.
21. Cross-border Rx: pharmaceutical manufacturers and U.S. international tax policy. Hearing Before the Committee on Finance, United States Senate. May 11, 2023.

Accessed January 26, 2024. https://www.finance.senate.gov/hearings/cross-border-rx-pharmaceutical-manufacturers-and-us-international-tax-policy.

22. Merelli A. Guess how much big pharma paid in US taxes on $110 billion of profit in 2022. Quartz. May 17, 2023. Accessed January 26, 2024. https://qz.com/guess-how-much-big-pharma-paid-in-us-taxes-on-110-bill-1850441135.
23. Dunleavy K. In his final full year as AbbVie's CEO, Richard Gonzalez collects $25.7M in total pay. Fierce Pharma. May 19, 2024. Accessed January 26, 2024. https://www.fiercepharma.com/pharma/his-final-full-year-abbvies-ceo-gonzalez-collects-257m#:~:text=In%20his%20final%20full%20year%20as%20AbbVie's%20CEO%2C%20Gonzalez%20collected,paid%20CEO%20in%20the%20industry.
24. Sanders B. Greedy pharma firms rip off Americans while Pfizer, Moderna swim in profits. Bernie Sanders. January 23, 2023. Accessed January 26, 2024. https://www.sanders.senate.gov/op-eds/greedy-pharma-firms-rip-off-americans-while-pfizer-moderna-swim-in-profits/#:~:text=Meanwhile%2C%20as%20Americans%20die%20because,in%20total%20compensation%20in%202021.
25. Meller A, Ahmed H. How big pharma reaps profits while hurting everyday Americans. Center for American Progress. August 30, 2019. Accessed January 26, 2024. https://www.americanprogress.org/article/big-pharma-reaps-profits-hurting-everyday-americans/#:~:text=As%20the%20report%20stated%2C%20%E2%80%9CAmong,margin%20across%20non%2Ddrug%20companies.
26. Stacciarini J. The global pharmaceutical sector: numbers and dynamics. Zenodo. 2024. https://doi.org/10.5281/zenodo.13891633.
27. Putterman S. Biden is right. The US generally pays double that of other countries for Rx drugs. KFF Health News. March 6, 2024. Accessed January 26, 2024. https://kffhealthnews.org/news/article/fact-check-biden-prescription-drug-prices-nation-comparison/.
28. Kurani N, Cotliar D, Cox C. How do prescription drug costs in the U.S. compare to other countries? Peterson-KFF Health System Tracker. February 8, 2022. Accessed January 27, 2024. Available at: https://www.healthsystemtracker.org/chart-collection/how-do-prescription-drug-costs-in-the-united-states-compare-to-other-countries/#Prices%20of%20select%20prescription%20drugs%20in%20the%20United%20States%20and%20for%20comparable%20countries,%202017.
29. McGregor N. Cost of care and physician responsibility. *NEJM Catalyst*. July 10, 2018. https://algorithms.utah.edu/blog/2018/03/nejm-cost-of-care.php.
30. Zhang Z. Harvard study: "cowboy doctors" partly to blame for healthcare costs. *Harvard Magazine*. August 11, 2015. Accessed January 27, 2024. https://www.harvardmagazine.com/2015/08/cowboy-doctors-and-health-costs.

31. Kannappan S, Darrow JJ, Kesselheim AS, Beall RF. The timing of 30-month stay expirations and generic entry: a cohort study of first generics, 2013-2020. *Clin Transl Sci.* 2021;14(5):1917-1923. https://doi.org/10.1111/cts.13046.
32. Guidance for Industry. 180-day exclusivity when multiple ANDAs are submitted on the same day. FDA. July 2003. https://www.fda.gov/media/71304/download#:~:text=During%20the%20exclusivity%20period%2C%20FDA,may%20approve%20all%20subsequent%20ANDAs. Accessed January 27, 2024.
33. Mailankody S, Prasad V. Five years of cancer drug approvals: innovation, efficacy, and costs. *JAMA Oncol.* 2015;1(4):539-540. doi:10.1001/jamaoncol.2015.0373
34. Medicare Prescription Drug, Improvement, and Modernization Act of 2003, Pub L No. 108-173, §1860D-11(i), 117 Stat 2066 (2003).
35. Medicare drug price negotiation program: understanding development and trends in utilization and spending for the selected drugs. ASPE Research Report. December 14, 2023. Accessed February 1, 2024. https://aspe.hhs.gov/sites/default/files/documents/4bf549a55308c3aadc74b34abcb7a1d1/ira-drug-negotiation-report.pdf.
36. Global oncology trends 2018. IQVIA Institute Report. May 24, 2018. Accessed February 1, 2024. https://www.iqvia.com/insights/the-iqvia-institute/reports/global-oncology-trends-2018.
37. Spurling GK, Mansfield PR, Montgomery BD, et al. Information from pharmaceutical companies and the quality, quantity, and cost of physicians' prescribing: a systematic review. *PLoS Med.* 2010;7(10):e1000352. doi:10.1371/journal.pmed.1000352
38. Abramson J. *Overdosed America: The Broken Promise of American Medicine.* New York: HarperCollins; 2005.

Chapter Three: How Sure Are You About Insurance?

1. Eltelbany M, Gattani R, Ofosu-Somuah A, Damluji A, Epps KC, Batchelor WB. Transcatheter PFO closure for cryptogenic stroke: current approaches and future considerations. *Front Cardiovasc Med.* 2024;11:1391886. https://doi.org/10.3389/fcvm.2024.1391886.
2. Fields R. How often do health insurers deny patients' claims? *ProPublica.* June 28, 2023. Accessed February 1, 2024. https://www.propublica.org/article/how-often-do-health-insurers-deny-patients-claims.
3. Armstrong D, Rucker P, Miller M. UnitedHealth healthcare tried to deny coverage to a chronically ill patient. He fought back, exposing the insurer's inner workings. *ProPublica.* February 2, 2023. Accessed February 1, 2024. https://www.propublica.org/article/unitedhealth-healthcare-insurance-denial-ulcerative-colitis.

4. Palosky C. Marketplace insurers denied nearly 1 in 5 in-network claims in 2020, though it's often not clear why. KFF News Release. July 5, 2022. Accessed February 9, 2023. https://www.kff.org/private-insurance/press-release/marketplace-insurers-denied-nearly-1-in-5-in-network-claims-in-2020-though-its-often-not-clear-why/.
5. Tolbert J, Damico A. Claims denials and appeals in ACA marketplace plans in 2024. Kaiser Family Foundation. 2024. Accessed April 3, 2026. https://www.kff.org/patient-consumer-protections/claims-denials-and-appeals-in-aca-marketplace-plans-in-2024/
6. Biniek JF, Sroczynski N, Freed M, Neuman T. Medicare Advantage plans denied 2 million prior authorization requests in 2021, about 6% of such requests. Kaiser Family Foundation. February 2, 2023. Accessed April 3, 2026. https://www.kff.org/medicare/press-release/medicare-advantage-plans-denied-2-million-prior-authorization-requests-in-2021-about-6-of-such-requests/
7. Pollitz K, Pestaina K, Lopes L, Wallace R, Lo J. Consumer problems with prior authorization: evidence from KFF survey. Kaiser Family Foundation. September 29, 2023. Accessed February 1, 2024. https://www.kff.org/affordable-care-act/issue-brief/consumer-problems-with-prior-authorization-evidence-from-kff-survey/.
8. Roy J. Your health insurance says, 'claim denied.' How to fight back. *The Los Angeles Times*. January 19, 2022. Accessed February 2, 2024. https://www.latimes.com/business/story/2022-01-19/how-to-appeal-an-insurance-claim-denial.
9. Berg S. What doctors wish patients knew about prior authorization. American Medical Association. September 11, 2023. Accessed February 2, 2024. https://www.ama-assn.org/practice-management/prior-authorization/what-doctors-wish-patients-knew-about-prior-authorization.
10. American Medical Association. 2024 AMA prior authorization (PA) physician survey. 2024. Accessed April 3, 2026. https://www.ama-assn.org/system/files/prior-authorization-survey.pdf
11. Sullivan L, Celik Z, Killelea A. Prior authorization reform heats up. Center on Health Insurance Reforms, Georgetown University. November 24, 2025. Accessed April 2, 2026. https://chir.georgetown.edu/prior-authorization-reform-heats-up/.
12. RCW 48.43.525. Prohibition against retrospective denial of health plan coverage—rules. Washington State Legislature. Accessed February 3, 2024. https://app.leg.wa.gov/rcw/default.aspx?cite=48.43.525.
13. 2023 employer health benefits survey: section 1. cost of health insurance. Kaiser Family Foundation. October 18, 2023. Accessed February 3, 2024. https://www.kff.org/report-section/ehbs-2023-section-1-cost-of-health-insurance/.

14. Mathews AW. Health insurance costs are taking the biggest jumps in years. *The Wall Street Journal.* Updated September 7, 2023. Accessed February 3, 2024. https://www.wsj.com/health/healthcare/health-insurance-cost-increase-5b35ead7.
15. Pearl R. Why health insurers can, but won't, break up medical monopolies. *Forbes.* March 13, 2023. Accessed February 4, 2024. https://www.forbes.com/sites/robertpearl/2023/03/13/why-health-insurers-can-but-wont-break-up-medical-monopolies/
16. Allen M. We asked prosecutors if health insurance companies care about fraud; they laughed at us. *ProPublica.* September 10, 2019. Accessed February 4, 2024. https://www.propublica.org/article/we-asked-prosecutors-if-health-insurance-companies-care-about-fraud-they-laughed-at-us.
17. Owens C. Major health insurance companies are nearing too big to fail status. Axios. April 19, 2024. Accessed February 4, 2024. https://www.axios.com/2024/04/19/health-insurance-companies-uhg-aetna-cigna.
18. Minhas A. Net income of UnitedHealth group from 2007 to 2023. Statista. March 3, 2026. Accessed April 3, 2026. https://www.statista.com/statistics/241026/total-revenue-of-unitedhealth/.
19. Merelli A. Fixing America's health insurance woes is 'actually very simple,' says leading economist. Stat News. October 23, 2023. Accessed February 4, 2024. https://www.statnews.com/2023/10/23/universal-health-care-amy-finkelstein/.
20. The White House. Fact sheet: President Donald J. Trump announces actions to make healthcare prices transparent. Published February 25, 2025. Accessed April 2, 2026. https://www.whitehouse.gov/fact-sheets/2025/02/fact-sheet-president-donald-j-trump-announces-actions-to-make-healthcare-prices-transparent/
21. Lo J, Claxton G. Wager E. Cox C, Amin K. Ongoing challenges with hospital price transparency. Kaiser Family Foundation. February 10, 2023. Accessed February 4, 2024. https://www.kff.org/health-costs/issue-brief/ongoing-challenges-with-hospital-price-transparency/.
22. Potter W. *Deadly Spin: An Insurance Company Insider Speaks Out on How Corporate PR Is Killing Health Care and Deceiving Americans.* New York, NY: Bloomsbury Press; 2010.

Chapter Four: Is Healthcare Any of Your Business?

1. Schulte F. Sick profit: investigating private equity's stealthy takeover of health care across cities and specialties. KFF Health News. November 14, 2022. Accessed February 4, 2024. https://kffhealthnews.org/news/article/private-equity-takeover-health-care-cities-specialties/.
2. Lee C. KFF's Kaiser Health News investigates private equity's stealth takeover of health care in the United States. KFF Press Release. November 14, 2022.

Accessed February 6, 2024. https://www.kff.org/health-costs/press-release/kffs-kaiser-health-news-investigates-private-equitys-stealth-takeover-of-health-care-in-the-united-states/.

3. America's Health Insurance Plans. Lower quality at higher costs. AHIP Private Equity Issue Brief. AHIP. September 15, 2022. Accessed February 6, 2024. https://www.ahip.org/resources/ahip-private-equity-issue-brief.
4. Blumenthal D. Private equity's role in health care. The Commonwealth Fund Explainer. November 17, 2023. Accessed February 6, 2024. https://www.commonwealthfund.org/publications/explainer/2023/nov/private-equity-role-health-care.
5. Bugbee M. How private equity has looted our hospitals—and what we can do to stop it. *AFT Health Care*. 2024;5(2). Accessed April 3, 2026. https://www.aft.org/hc/fall2024/bugbee.
6. Scheffler RM, Alexander L, Fulton BD, Arnold DR, Abdelhadi OA. Monetizing medicine: private equity and competition in physician practice markets. American Trust Institute. July 10, 2023. Accessed February 8, 2024. https://www.antitrustinstitute.org/wp-content/uploads/2023/07/AAI-UCB-EG_Private-Equity-I-Physician-Practice-Report_FINAL.pdf.
7. Weil J. The private equity deal that flattened a hospital chain and its landlord. *The Wall Street Journal*. May 7, 2024. Accessed August 8, 2024. https://www.wsj.com/finance/the-private-equity-deal-that-flattened-a-hospital-chain-and-its-landlord-3096747d.
8. Borsa A, Bejarano G, Ellen M, Bruch JD. Evaluating trends in private equity ownership and impacts on health outcomes, costs, and quality: systematic review. *BMJ*. 2023;382:e075244. Accessed February 8, 2024. https://doi.org/10.1136/bmj-2023-075244.
9. Kannan S, Bruch JD, Song Z. Changes in hospital adverse events and patient outcomes associated with private equity acquisition. *JAMA*. 2023;330(24):2365-2375. Accessed February 8, 2024. https://doi.org/10.1001/jama.2023.23147.
10. Regulatory overload: assessing the regulatory burden on health systems, hospitals and post-acute care providers. American Hospital Association. October 2017. Accessed February 8, 2024. https://www.aha.org/sites/default/files/regulatory-overload-report.pdf.
11. Nguyen KL. HIPAA: at what cost? *Medical Economics*. September 9, 2019. Accessed February 9, 2024. https://www.medicaleconomics.com/view/hipaa-what-cost.
12. Kane CK. Recent changes in physician practice arrangements: shifts away from private practice and towards larger practice size continue through 2022. Policy Research Perspective. Chicago: American Medical Association; 2023. Accessed February 9, 2024. https://www.ama-assn.org/system/files/2022-prp-practice-arrangement.pdf.

13. Muoio D. Federal regulators, clinicians make their case against private equity in healthcare. Fierce Healthcare. March 6, 2024. Accessed April 9, 2024. https://www.fiercehealthcare.com/regulatory/federal-regulators-clinicians-make-their-case-against-private-equity-healthcare.
14. Karas LO. The private equity takeover of medicine. *The Systemic Justice Journal.* Vol. 1. Accessed February 11, 2024. https://systemicjustice.org/article/the-private-equity-takeover-of-medicine/.
15. Jacoby D, Herschman G. Why so many physicians are partnering with private equity. *Medical Economics.* June 20, 2023. Accessed February 11, 2024. https://www.medicaleconomics.com/view/why-so-many-physicians-are-partnering-with-private-equity.
16. Zhu JM, Zeveney A, Read S. Crowley R. Physician perspectives on private equity investment in health care. *JAMA Intern Med.* 2024;184(5):579-580. Accessed February 11, 2024. https://doi.org/10.1001/jamainternmed.2024.0062
17. Cornbrooks A. Physicians say practice ownership by non-physician organizations worsened patients' quality of care. Press Release. Physicians Advocacy Institute. December 4, 2023. Accessed February 11, 2024. https://www.physiciansadvocacyinstitute.org/Portals/0/assets/docs/PAI-Research/NORC-Employed-Physicians-Survey-Press-Release-FINAL-for-PAI.pdf?ver=FnkmJ6_1eO4YyNIPksOGog%3D%3D.
18. Khan LM. Remarks at the Private Capital, Public Impact Workshop on Private Equity in Healthcare. March 5, 2024. Accessed February 11, 2024. https://www.ftc.gov/system/files/ftc_gov/pdf/2024.03.05-chair-khan-remarks-at-the-private-capital-public-impact-workshop-on-private-equity-in-healthcare.pdf.
19. Code of ethics. National Association for Healthcare Quality. Accessed February 11, 2024. https://nahq.org/about-nahq/code-of-ethics/.
20. Code of ethics. American College of Healthcare Executives. Accessed February 11, 2024. https://www.ache.org/about-ache/our-story/our-commitments/ethics/ache-code-of-ethics.
21. National dental management company pays $24 million to resolve fraud allegations. Press Release. U.S. Department of Justice. January 20, 2010. February 11, 2024. https://www.justice.gov/opa/pr/national-dental-management-company-pays-24-million-resolve-fraud-allegations.
22. Domino D. Small Smiles agrees to $39M settlement in mistreatment lawsuit. DrBicuspid.com. May 11, 2015. Accessed February 11, 2024. https://www.drbicuspid.com/dental-specialties/pediatrics/article/15370743/small-smiles-agrees-to-39m-settlement-in-mistreatment-lawsuit.
23. $39 million available to Small Smiles Dental Center Patients—providing approval by court. Dentist the Menace blog. May 6, 2015. Accessed February 11, 2024. https://blog.dentistthemenace.com/2015/05/39-million-available-to-small-smiles.html.

24. Braun RT, Bond AM, Qian Y, Zhang M, Casalino LP. Private Equity In Dermatology: Effect On Price, Utilization, And Spending. Health Aff (Millwood). 2021 May;40(5):727-735. doi: 10.1377/hlthaff.2020.02062. PMID: 33939519.
25. Sinclair U. *The Jungle*. New York: Doubleday, Page & Company; 1906.
26. National Labor Relations Act, 29 U.S.C. §§ 151–169 (1935).

Part Two: How Your Doctor Became a Pawn

1. Bailey R. The case of Dr. Anna Pou—physician liability in emergency situations. *Virtual Mentor*. 2010;12(9):726–730. https://doi.org/10.1001/virtualmentor.2010.12.9.hlaw1-1009.
2. Fink S. The deadliest storm. *N Y Times Magazine*. August 30, 2009. Accessed February 11, 2024. https://www.nytimes.com/2009/08/30/magazine/30doctors.html
3. Simons R. 'Five Days at Memorial': what happened to Dr. Anna Pou and where is she now? *Newsweek*. August 12, 2022. Accessed February 12, 2024. https://www.newsweek.com/five-days-memorial-apple-tv-plus-what-happened-dr-anna-pou-where-she-now-1732451.

Chapter Five: Your Doctor Is Also Struggling (The Doctor's View)

1. Guardado JR. Medical liability claim frequency among U.S. physicians. *American Medical Association Policy Research Perspectives*. April 2023. Accessed February 12, 2024. https://www.ama-assn.org/system/files/policy-research-perspective-medicalliability-claim-frequency.pdf.
2. Vizcaino-Rakosnik M, Martin-Fumado C, Arimany-Manso J, Gomez-Duran E. The impact of malpractice claims on physicians' well-being and practice. *J. Patient Saf.* 2022; 18(1):46-51. https://doi.org/10.1097/pts.0000000000000800
3. JAMA and Archives Journals. Many U.S. physicians believe their own patients are receiving too much care, survey shows. *ScienceDaily*. September 26, 2011. Accessed February 13, 2024.www.sciencedaily.com/releases/2011/09/110926165911.htm.
4. Woolhandler S, Himmelstein DU. Administrative work consumes one-sixth of U.S. physicians' working hours and lowers their career satisfaction. *Int J Health Serv.* 2014;44(4):635-642. https://doi.org/10.2190/hs.44.4.a.
5. Lane K. Physician compensation report 2018. Medscape. April 11, 2018. Accessed February 12, 2024. https://www.medscape.com/slideshow/2018-compensation-overview-6009667.
6. Porter J, Boyd C, Skandari MR, Laiteerapong N. Revisiting the time needed to provide adult primary care. *J Gen Intern Med.* 2023;38: 147–155. https://doi.org/10.1007/s11606-022-07707-x

7. Spoehr C. New AAMC report shows continuing projected physician shortage. AAMC Press Release. March 21, 2024. Accessed February 12, 2024. https://www.aamc.org/news/press-releases/new-aamc-report-shows-continuing-projected-physician-shortage
8. Shanafelt TD, Dyrbye LN, West CP, Wang H, Carlasare LE, *et al.* Career plans of US physicians after the first 2 years of the COVID 19 pandemic. *Mayo Clin Proc.* 2023;98(11):1629-1640. https://doi.org/10.1016/j.mayocp.2023.07.006.
9. Rosenthal E. The shrinking number of primary care physicians is reaching a tipping point. KFF Health News Perspective. September 8, 2023. Accessed February 13, 2024. https://kffhealthnews.org/news/article/lack-of-primary-care tipping-point/.
10. Association of American Medical Colleges. The complexities of physician supply and demand: projections from 2021 to 2036. 2023. Accessed February 13, 2024. https://www.aamc.org/media/75236/download.
11. U.S. Department of Health and Human Services. Access to health services. Healthy People 2030. Accessed February 13, 2024. https://odphp.health.gov/healthypeople/priority-areas/social-determinants-health/literature-summaries/access-health-services.
12. Paavola A. Unnecessary ER visits cost $47B a year, report finds. *Becker's Hospital Review.* October 1, 2021. Accessed February 13, 2024. https://www.beckershospitalreview.com/finance/unnecessary-er-visits-cost-47b-a-year-report-finds.html#:~:text=Unnecessary%20emergency%20room%20visits%20caused,consulting%20and%20IT%20firm%20Accenture.
13. Health Maintenance Organization Act of 1973, Pub L No. 93-222, 87 Stat 914 (1973).
14. Hawkes N. The role of NHS gatekeeping in delayed diagnosis. *BMJ.* 2014;348:g2633 https://doi.org/10.1136/bmj.g2633.
15. Spivack SB, Murray GF, Lewis VA. A decade of ACOs in Medicare: have they delivered on their promise? *J Health Polit Policy Law.* 2023;48(1):63-90. https://doi.org/10.1215/03616878-10171090.
16. AAFP. Accountable care organizations: answers to common questions. AAFP. https://www.aafp.org/family-physician/practice-and-career/delivery-payment-models/acos.html.
17. What is pay for performance in healthcare? *NEJM Catalyst.* March 1, 2018. https://catalyst.nejm.org/doi/full/10.1056/CAT.18.0245
18. Measuring and addressing physician burnout. American Medical Association. Updated May 15, 2025. Accessed February 15, 2024. https://www.ama-assn.org/practice-management/physician-health/measuring-and-addressing-physician-burnout#:~:text=The%20most%20recent%20study%20in,up%20from%2038%25%20in%202020.

19. Burn-out: an occupational phenomenon. World Health Organization. Accessed February 15, 2024. https://www.who.int/standards/classifications/frequently-asked-questions/burn-out-an-occupational-phenomenon#:~:text=It%20is%20characterized%20by%20three,reduced%20professional%20efficacy.
20. Talbot SG, Dean W. Physicians aren't 'burning out.' they are suffering from moral injury. *STAT*. July 26, 2018. Accessed February 15, 2024. https://www.statnews.com/2018/07/26/physicians-not-burning-out-they-are-suffering-moral-injury/.
21. Dean W, Talbot S, Dean A. Reframing clinician distress: moral injury not burnout. *Fed Pract.* 2019;36(9):400-402. Erratum in: *Fed Pract.* 2019;36(10):447. PMID: 31571807; PMCID: PMC6752815.
22. Matheson J. Physician suicide. American College of Emergency Physicians. Accessed February 15, 2024. https://www.acep.org/life-as-a-physician/wellness/wellness/wellness-week-articles/physician-suicide.
23. Symon R. *Do No Harm*. Movie; 2018.
24. Dr. Lorna Breen Health Care Provider Protection Act, Pub L No. 117-105, 136 Stat 112 (2022).

Chapter Six: Who Defines the Standard of Care? (Competence)

1. Knowles E. Calculating delayed diagnosis damages. The Knowles Group blog. March 13, 2023. Accessed February 17, 2024. https://www.theknowlesgroup.org/blog/calculating-delayed-diagnosis-damages/.
2. Bieber C. Medical malpractice statistics. *Forbes*. January 25, 2024. Accessed February 17, 2024. https://www.forbes.com/advisor/legal/personal-injury/medical-malpractice-statistics/#:~:text=One%20in%20three%20care%20providers,medical%20malpractice%20during%20their%20care.&text=Care%20providers%20make%20avoidable%20errors,15%25%20of%20all%20medical%20interventions.&text=Misdiagnosis%20is%20one%20of%20the,most%20likely%20to%20be%20misdiagnosed.
3. Mills RJ. AMA: One in three physicians has been sued in their career. American Medical Association Press Release. May 10, 2023. Accessed February 17, 2024. https://www.ama-assn.org/press-center/press-releases/ama-one-three-physicians-previously-sued-their-career.
4. AMA studies show continued cost burden of the medical liability system. American Medical Association Press Release. January 24, 2018. Accessed February 17, 2024. https://www.ama-assn.org/press-center/press-releases/ama-studies-show-continued-cost-burden-medical-liability-system.
5. Bono MJ, Wermuth HR, Hipskind JE. Medical malpractice. In: StatPearls [Internet]. Florida: StatPearls Publishing; October 31, 2022. Accessed February 17, 2024. https://www.ncbi.nlm.nih.gov/books/NBK470573/.

6. Frakes M. Defensive medicine and obstetric practices. *J Empir Legal Studies*. 2012;9(3).
7. Popowitz E. Addressing the healthcare staffing shortage. Definitive Healthcare. 2023. Accessed February 18, 2024. https://www.definitivehc.com/resources/research/healthcare-staffing-shortage.
8. Cocchiarale F, Gnatowski M Jr, Pensa G. Medical malpractice stress syndrome. *Emerg Med Clin North Am*. 2025;43(1):1-7. https://doi.org/10.1016/j.emc.2024.05.024.
9. Jarry J. Medical error is not the third leading cause of death. McGill University. August 27, 2021. Accessed February 18, 2024. https://www.mcgill.ca/oss/article/critical-thinking-health/medical-error-not-third-leading-cause-death.
10. Mello MM, Chandra A, Gawande AA, Studdert DM. National costs of the medical liability system. *Health Aff (Millwood)*. 2010;29(9):1569-1577. https://doi.org/10.1377/hlthaff.2009.0807.
11. Medical liability premiums: trends and analysis. American Medical Association. Accessed February18, 2024. https://www.ama-assn.org/system/files/prp-mlm-premiums-2021.pdf.
12. Birkhauer J, Gaab J, Kossowsky J, Hasler S, Krummenacher P, Werner C, Gerger H. Trust in the health care professional and health outcome: a meta-analysis. *PloSOne*. 2017;12(2):e0170988. https://doi.org/10.1371/journal.pone.0170988
13. Pear A. Medical malpractice: a missed opportunity in health care. *The New York Times*. May 27, 2019. Accessed February 20, 2024.https://www.nytimes.com/2019/05/27/upshot/malpractice-health-care-missed-opportunity.html.
14. Gawande A. *The Checklist Manifesto: How to Get Things Right*. New York: Metropolitan Books; 2009.
15. Mukherjee S. Surgical checklists save lives—but once in a while, they don't. Why? *The New York Times Magazine*. May 9, 2018. https://www.nytimes.com/2018/05/09/magazine/surgical-checklists-save-lives-but-once-in-a-while-they-dont-why.html.

Chapter Seven: Are We Beholden to Our Electronic Mistresses? (Access)

1. Rajaee L. The history of electronic health records (EHRs). Elation Health blog. November 7, 2025. Accessed April 3, 2026. https://www.elationhealth.com/resources/blogs/the-history-of-electronic-health-records-ehrs.
2. Atherton J. Development of the electronic health record. *Virtual Mentor*. 2011;13(3):186-189. https://doi.org/10.1001/virtualmentor.2011.13.3.mhst1-1103.

3. Evans RS. Electronic health records: then, now, and in the future. *Yearb Med Inform*. 2016;(Suppl1):S48-S61. https://doi.org/10.15265/IYS-2016-s006.
4. Voltz D. The rise of EMR innovators and explorers. HIT Consultant. September 3, 2014. Accessed February 20, 2024. https://hitconsultant.net/2014/09/03/the-rise-of-emr-innovators-and-explorers/.
5. Burde H. HITECH Act: an overview. *Virtual Mentor*. 2011;13(3):172-175. https://doi.org/10.1001/virtualmentor.2011.13.3.hlaw1-1103.
6. Alammari D, Banta JE, Shah H. Reibling E, Ramadan M. Meaningful use of electronic health records and ambulatory healthcare quality measures. *Cureus*. 2021;13(1):e13036. https://doi.org/10.7759/cureus.13036.
7. Jercich K. Hospital EHR spending projected to reach $99B by 2024. Healthcare IT News. May 21, 2020. Accessed February 22, 2024. https://www.healthcareitnews.com/news/hospital-ehr-spending-projected-reach-99b-2024.
8. Electronic health records fail to detect 33% of medication errors. University of Utah Press Release. May 29, 2020. Accessed February 22, 2024. https://healthcare.utah.edu/press-releases/2020/05/electronic-health-records-fail-detect33-of-medication-errors.
9. Krevat SA, Samuel S, Boxley C, Mohan V, Siegal D, *et al.* Identifying electronic health record contributions to diagnostic error in ambulatory settings through legal claims analysis. *JAMA Netw Open*. 2023;6(4):e238399. https://doi.org/10.1001/jamanetworkopen.2023.8399.
10. Thompson G, O'Horo JC, Pickering BW, Herasevich V. Impact of the electronic medical record on mortality, length of stay, and cost in the hospital and ICU. *Crit Care Med*. 2015;43(6). Accessed February 22, 2024. https://doi.org/10.1097/CCM.0000000000000948.
11. DiGiorgio AM, Mummaneni PV. Death by 10,000 clicks: the electronic health record. MedPage Today. January 21, 2023. Accessed February 22, 2024. https://www.medpagetoday.com/opinion/second-opinions/102722.
12. Yanamadala S, Morrison D, Curtin C, McDonald K, Hernandez-Boussard T. Electronic health records and quality of care: an observational study modeling impact on mortality, readmissions, and complications. *Medicine (Baltimore)*. 2016;95(19):e3332. https://doi.org/10.1097/MD.0000000000003332.
13. Campanella P, Lovato E, Marone C, Fallacara L, Mancuso A, *et al.* The impact of electronic health records on healthcare quality: a systematic review and meta-analysis. *Eur J Public Health*. 2016;26(1):60-64. https://doi.org/10.1093/eurpub/ckv122.
14. ISMP resources for medication safety. ECRI. https://home.ecri.org/blogs/ismp-resources. Accessed February 22, 2024.
15. Urban H. It's time to expect more from EHRs. *Medical Economics*. July 6, 2023. Accessed February 24, 2024. https://www.medicaleconomics.com/view/it-s-time-to-expect-more-from-ehrs.

16. Phillips L. Healthcare cybersecurity in 2023: Hive's shutdown is good news but cyberattacks are only getting worse. eMarketer. July 27, 2023. Accessed February 24, 2024. https://www.emarketer.com/content/healthcare-cybersecurity-2023-hive-s-shutdown-good-news-cyberattacks-only-getting-worse.
17. Everson J, Adler-Milstein J. Gaps in health information exchange between hospitals that treat many shared patients. *J Am Med Inform Assoc.* 2018;25(9):1114-1121. https://doi.org/10.1093/jamia/ocy089.
18. Stanford Medicine. Doctors call for overhaul of electronic health records. *PR Newswire.* Published June 4, 2018. Accessed February 24, 2024. https://www.prnewswire.com/news-releases/doctors-call-for-overhaul-of-electronic-health-records-300659100.html
19. Brusie C. New study predicts a mass exodus of healthcare workers by 2025. Nurse.org. March 22, 2022. Accessed February 24, 2024. https://nurse.org/articles/healthcare-workers-leaving-2025/.
20. Smith T. Who are the largest EHR vendors? EHR in Practice. Accessed February 24, 2024. Updated October 31, 2025. https://www.ehrinpractice.com/largest-ehr-vendors.html.
21. Tate C, Warburton P. US hospital EMR market share 2019. KLAS Research. April 30, 2019. Accessed February 24, 2024. https://klasresearch.com/report/us-hospital-emr-market-share-2019-significant-movement-in-every-market-sector/1454.
22. Bruce G. Epic's revenue by year. *Becker's Hospital Review*. December 1, 2023. Accessed February 24, 2024. https://www.beckershospitalreview.com/ehrs/epics-revenue-by-year.html.
23. Bruce G. Epic's dominance in 12 numbers. *Becker's Hospital Review*. July 18, 2024. Accessed April 2, 2026. https://www.beckershospitalreview.com/healthcare-information-technology/ehrs/epics-dominance-in-12-numbers/.
24. Jennings K. The billionaire who controls your medical records. *Forbes*. April 8, 2021. Accessed February 25, 2024. https://www.forbes.com/sites/katiejennings/2021/04/08/billionaire-judy-faulkner-epic-systems/?sh=66639553575a.
25. What practices look for when selecting EHR (2022 EHR Report). Software Path. January 18, 2022. Accessed February 25, 2024. https://softwarepath.com/guides/ehr-report.
26. Japsen B. Doctor practices still reeling from loss of support staff since pandemic's beginning. *Forbes*. September 1, 2023. Accessed February 25, 2024. https://www.forbes.com/sites/brucejapsen/2023/09/01/doctor-practices-still-reeling-from-loss-of-support-staff-since-pandemics-beginning/?sh=421302a36a5e.
27. Brown SH, Lincoln MJ, Groen PJ, Kolodner RM. VistA—U.S. Department of Veterans Affairs national-scale HIS. *Int J Med Inform*. 2003;69(2-3):135-156. https://doi.org/10.1016/S1386-5056(02)00150-1.

28. Meagher E. Time for VA to admit EHR system is a failure, revert back to VistA. Federal News Network. May 10, 2023. Accessed February 25, 2024. https://federalnewsnetwork.com/commentary/2023/05/time-for-va-to-admit-the-ehr-system-is-a-failure-revert-back-to-vista/.
29. Diaz N. VA links 4 deaths to its Oracle Cerner EHR system. *Becker's Hospital Review*. March 16, 2023. Accessed February 25, 2024. https://www.beckershospitalreview.com/ehrs/va-says-4-deaths-linked-to-its-oraclecerner-ehr-system.html.
30. Reisman M. EHRs: the challenge of making electronic data usable and interoperable. PT. 2017;42(9):572-575. https://pubmed.ncbi.nlm.nih.gov/28890644/.
31. Adler-Milstein J, Pfeifer E. Information blocking: is it occurring and what policy strategies can address it? *Millbank Q*. 2017;95(1):117-135. https://doi.org/10.1111/1468-0009.12247.
32. Sinsky C, Colligan L, Li L, Prgomet M, Reynolds S, *et al*. Allocation of physician time in ambulatory practice: a time and motion study in 4 specialties. *Ann Intern Med*. 2016;165(11): 753-760. https://doi.org/10.7326/m16-0961.
33. Promoting Interoperability Programs. CMS.gov. Accessed February 26, 2024. https://www.cms.gov/medicare/regulations-guidance/promoting-interoperability-programs.
34. Shem S. *Man's 4th Best Hospital*. New York: HarperCollins; 2004.

Chapter Eight: Have We Been Legislated Out? (Incentives)

1. False Claims Act. Civil Division, U.S. Department of Justice. Accessed February 28, 2024. https://www.justice.gov/civil/false-claims-act.
2. False Claims Act settlements and judgments exceed $2 billion in fiscal year 2022. U.S. Department of Justice Press Release. February 7, 2023. Accessed February 28, 2024. https://www.justice.gov/opa/pr/false-claimsact-settlements-and-judgments-exceed-2-billion-fiscal-year-2022.
3. 2020 estimated improper payment rates for Centers for Medicare & Medicaid Services (CMS) programs. CMS.gov. November 16, 2020. Accessed February 28, 2024. https://www.cms.gov/newsroom/fact-sheets/2020-estimated-improper-payment-rates-centers-medicare-medicaid-services-cms-programs.
4. Verhovshek J. Under coding is no better than over coding. AAPC blog. April 4, 2014. Accessed February 28, 2024. https://www.aapc.com/blog/26957-undercoding-is-no-better-than-overcoding/.
5. Fraud and abuse laws. Office of Inspector General, U.S. Department of Health and Human Services. Accessed March 1, 2024. https://oig.hhs.gov/compliance/physician-education/fraud-abuse-laws/.

6. Constantine Cannon. Anti-kickback statute and Stark law. Constantine Cannon. Accessed March 1, 2024. https://constantinecannon.com/practice/whistleblower/whistleblower-types/healthcare-fraud/anti-kickback-stark/.
7. Physician-owned hospitals. CMS.org. Accessed March 1, 2024. https://www.cms.gov/medicare/regulations-guidance/physician-self-referral/physician-owned-hospitals.
8. FY 2024 hospital inpatient prospective payment system (IPPS) and long-term care hospital prospective payment system. CMS.org. March 1, 2024. https://www.cms.gov/newsroom/fact-sheets/fy-2024-hospital-inpatient-prospective-payment-system-ipps-and-long-term-care-hospital-prospective. Accessed
9. Plummer E, Cram P, Bai G. Who's afraid of physician-owned hospitals? *MedPage Today*. July 6, 2023. Accessed March 1, 2024. https://www.medpagetoday.com/opinion/second-opinions/105351.
10. Wang Y, Plummer E, Wang Y, Cram P, Bai G. Comparison of commercial negotiated price and cash price between physician-owned hospitals and other hospitals in the same hospital referral region. *JAMA Netw Open*. 2023;6(6):e2319980. Accessed March 2, 2024. https://doi.org/10.1001/jamanetworkopen.2023.19980.
11. Hagland M. MD-owned hospitals: is a policy debate being overshadowed by financial troubles? Healthcare Innovation blog. August 31, 2023. Accessed March 2, 2024. https://www.hcinnovationgroup.com/policy-value-based-care/medicare-medicaid/blog/53072080/md-owned-hospitals-is-a-policy-debate-being-overshadowed-by-financial-troubles.
12. Stanger K. Requiring referrals from employees and contractors. Holland & Hart LLP. December 19, 2016. Accessed March 2, 2024. https://www.hollandhart.com/requiring-referrals-from-employees-and-contractors.
13. Feldman M. Unintended consequences of perfectly good programs and policies. *MDedge Rheumatology*. January 18, 2023. Accessed March 2, 2024. https://csro.info/UserFiles/file/Unintendedconsequencesof_MDedgeRheumatology.pdf.
14. Cowart H. How physicians accidentally violate the Stark Law. Hendershot Cowart PC blog. January 2, 2018. Accessed March 2, 2024. https://www.hchlawyers.com/blog/2018/january/how-physicians-accidentally-violate-the-stark-la/.
15. Centers for Medicare & Medicaid Services. *Modernizing and clarifying the physician self-referral regulations (Stark Law) and the Anti-Kickback Statute (AKS): final rule*. Fed Regist. 2020;85(232):77492-77679.
16. American Medical Association. Protecting the patient-physician relationship: issue brief. Accessed March 4, 2024. https://www.ama-assn.org/system/files/protecting-patient-physician-relationship-issue-brief.pdf.

17. Martins L, Schweikart S. Physician free speech and the doctor-patient relationship post-Dobbs. The Petrie-Flom Center blog. May 25, 2023. Accessed March 4, 2024. https://blog.petrieflom.law.harvard.edu/2023/05/25/physician-free-speech-and-the-doctor-patient-relationship-post-dobbs/.
18. Office of Inspector General, US Department of Health and Human Services. Fraud and abuse; removal of safe harbor protection for rebates involving prescription pharmaceuticals and creation of new safe harbors; final rule. *Fed Regist.* 2020;85(232):77684-77801.
19. Cronin AJ. *The Citadel.* London, UK: Victor Gollancz Ltd; 1937.
20. The National Health Service: A Political History. Webster C. *The National Health Service: A Political History.* 2nd ed. Oxford University Press; 2002.

Part Three: Toward Building a Better System

1. Merschel M. The presidential heart attack that changed America. American Heart Association. February 15, 2024. Accessed March 5, 2024. https://www.heart.org/en/news/2024/02/15/the-presidential-heart-attack-that-changed-america.
2. Rakshit S, Winger A, Cotter L, McGough M, Wager E, Cox C. How has U.S. spending on healthcare changed over time? Peterson-KFF Health System Tracker. January 22, 2026. Accessed March 5, 2024. https://www.healthsystemtracker.org/chart-collection/u-s-spending-healthcare-changed-time/.
3. Tikkanen R, Abrams MK. U.S. health care from a global perspective: 2019. The Commonwealth Fund Issue Brief. January 30, 2020. Accessed March 5, 2024. https://www.commonwealthfund.org/publications/issue-briefs/2020/jan/us-health-care-global-perspective-2019#:~:text=A%202015%20Commonwealth%20Fund%20brief,to%20other%20high%2Dincome%20countries.
4. How relevant is the American Medical Association? The Health Care Blog. June 20, 2009. Accessed March 5, 2024. Available at: https://thehealthcareblog.com/blog/2009/06/20/how-relevant-is-the-american-medical-association/.

Chapter Nine: The Intimacy Gap

1. Wikipedia contributors. *Aequanimitas.* Wikipedia. January 24, 2026, 05:33 UTC. Accessed March 5, 2024. https://en.wikipedia.org/w/index.php?title=Aequanimitas&oldid=1334549180.
2. Gutheil TG, Simon RI. Non-sexual boundary crossings and boundary violations: the ethical dilemma. *Psychiatr Clin North Am.* 2002;25(3):585-592. February 23, 2024. https://doi.org/10.1016/s0193-953x(01)00012-0.
3. Fox We, Fraher E, Huffstetler A, Moore D, Isasi F, Knestrick J. Health is primary: charting a path to equity and sustainability. *PCC Annual Evidence Report.* October 26, 2023. Accessed March 5, 2024. https://thepcc.org/sites/default

/files/resources/pcc-evidence-report-2023.pdf?utm_source=bitly&utm_medium=link&utm_campaign=2023_evidence.

4. AAMC. Total physicians by specialty, United States and its territories. Accessed February 13, 2024. https://www.aamc.org/data-reports/report/us-physician-workforce-data-dashboard.
5. Coodley G. The demise of primary care in America. KevinMD. December 20, 2022. Accessed March 7, 2024. https://www.kevinmd.com/2022/12/the-demise-of-primary-care-in-america.html.
6. Rao A, Shi Z, Ray KN, Mehrotra A, Ganguli I. National trends in primary care visit use and practice capabilities, 2008-2015. *Ann Fam Med.* 2019;17(6):538-544. Accessed March 7, 2024. https://doi.org/10.1370/afm.2474.
7. Kao H, Conant R, Soriano T, McCormick W. The past, present, and future of house calls. *Clin Geriatric Med.* 2009;25(1):19-34. Accessed March 7, 2024. https://www.geriatric.theclinics.com/article/S0749-0690(08)00063-3/abstract.
8. Rhyan CN. Travel and wait times are longest for health care services and result in an annual opportunity cost of $89 billion. *Altarum Research Brief.* Accessed March 7, 2024. https://altarum.org/news-and-insights/travel-and-wait-times-are-longest-health-care-services-and-result-annual.
9. Overhage JM, McCallie D. Physician time spent using the electronic health record during outpatient encounters: a descriptive study. *Ann Intern Med.* 2020;172(3):169-174. Accessed March 7, 2024. https://doi.org/10.7326/m18-3684.
10. Toscano F, O'Donnell E, Broderick JE, May M, Tucker P, Unruh MA, et al. How physicians spend their work time: an ecological momentary assessment. *J Gen Intern Med.* 2020;35(11):3166-3172. https://doi.org/10.1007/s11606-020-06087-4.
11. Rosen A. Using an EMR in front of a patient is akin to distracted driving. Doximity. September 30, 2019. Accessed March 7, 2024. https://opmed.doximity.com/articles/using-an-emr-in-front-of-a-patient-is-akin-to-distracted-driving.
12. Looking at electronic health records diverts doctors' attention from patients during office visits. News-Medical. January 24, 2014. Accessed March 7, 2024. https://www.news-medical.net/news/20140124/Looking-at-electronic-health-records-diverts-doctorsattention-from-patients-during-office-visits.aspx.
13. Maslach C, Jackson SE, Leiter MP. *Maslach Burnout Inventory Manual.* 3rd ed. Palo Alto, CA: Consulting Psychologists Press; 1996.
14. James TA. Building empathy into the structure of health care. Harvard Medical School. January 12, 2023. Accessed March 7, 2024. https://postgraduateeducation.hms.harvard.edu/trends-medicine/building-empathy

-structure-health-care#:~:text=Studies%20demonstrate%20how%20 empathy%20improves,they%20feel%20heard%20and%20understood.

15. Dastres J. Let's talk about nonsexual emotional and physical intimacy. Ships blog. Accessed March 8, 2024. https://www.shipspsychology.com.au/blog/nonsexual -emotional-and-physical-intimacy.
16. Adams P. *Gesundheit!: Bringing Good Health to You, the Medical System, and Society Through Physician Service, Complementary Therapies, Humor, and Joy*. Rochester, VT: Healing Arts Press; 1998.
17. Patch Adams. Accessed March 8, 2024. https://www.patchadams.org/.
18. Baker, A. *Crossing the Quality Chasm: A New Health System for the 21st Century*. BMJ;2001. Accessed March 8, 2024. https://doi.org/10.1136/bmj.323.7322 .1192.

Chapter Ten: The Magic of Shared Storytelling

1. Bernstein E. Why good storytellers are happier in life and in love. *The Wall Street Journal*. July 4, 2016. Accessed March 9, 2024. https://www.wsj.com/articles /why-good-storytellers-are-happier-in-life-and-in-love-1467652052.
2. Yang Y, Liu D, Liu B, Ou W, Want L, Ma Y, et al. Prevalence of post-traumatic stress disorder status among healthcare workers and its impact on their mental health during the crisis of COVID-19: a cross-sectional study. *Front Public Health*. 2022;10:904550. Accessed March 9, 2024. https://doi.org/10.3389/fpubh.2022 .904550.
3. Oi G, Yuan P, Qi M, Hu X, Shi S, Shi X. Influencing factors of high PTSD among medical staff during COVID-19: evidences from both meta-analysis and subgroup analysis. *Saf Health Work*. 2022;13(3):269-278. Accessed March 9, 2024. https://doi.org/10.1016/j.shaw.2022.06.003
4. Hu YY, Fix ML, Hervelone ND, Lipsitz SR, Greenberg CC, Weissman JS, Shapiro J. Physicians' needs in coping with emotional stressors: the case for peer support. *Arch Surg*. 2011;147(3):212-217. Accessed March 9, 2024. https://doi.org/10 .1001/archsurg.2011.312.
5. Busch IM, Moretti F, Purgato M, Barbui C, Wu A, Rimondini M. Psychological and psychosomatic symptoms of second victims of adverse events: a systemic review and meta-analysis. *J Patient Saf*. 2019;16(2):61-74. Accessed March 9, 2024. https://doi.org/10.1097/PTS.0000000000000589.
6. Grumet J. An apology. April 8, 2011; Grumet J. Broken. September 3, 2010. *Pulse: Voices from the Heart of Medicine*. https://pulsevoices.org/?s=Grumet.
7. Narrative exposure therapy. American Psychological Association. Accessed March 9, 2024. https://www.apa.org/ptsd-guideline/treatments/narrative -exposure-therapy.

8. Narrative medicine: patient panels. University of Washington Department of Dermatology. April 25, 2023. Accessed March 10, 2024. https://derm.uw.edu/news/narrative-medicine-patient-panels-combat-bias-burnout-through-storytelling.
9. Thoele DG, Gunalp C, Baran D, Harris J, Moss D, Donovan R, Li Y, Getz MA. Health Care Practitioners and Families Writing Together: The Three-Minute Mental Makeover. *Perm J*. 2020;24:19. Accessed March 10, 2024. https://doi.org/10.7812/TPP/19.056.
10. Pearl R. Physician burnout, isolation, and the erosion of the doctor-patient relationship. *Forbes*. August 12, 2019. Accessed March 10, 2026. https://www.forbes.com/sites/robertpearl/2019/08/12/physician-burnout-isolation/
11. Dias J, Hammill J. What is allyship? Your questions answered. Center for Creative Leadership. November 3, 2024. Accessed March 10, 2024. https://www.ccl.org/articles/leading-effectively-articles/what-is-allyship-your-questions-answered/.
12. McAbee J. Understanding stakeholder theory. Wrike blog. June 1, 2022. Accessed March 10, 2024. https://www.wrike.com/blog/understanding-stakeholder-theory/.
13. Storytelling leadership: how to use stories and narratives to communicate and persuade your audience and stakeholders. FasterCapital. April 4, 2025. Accessed March 10, 2026. https://fastercapital.com/content/Storytelling-Leadership--How-to-Use-Stories-and-Narratives-to-Communicate-and-Persuade-Your-Audience-and-Stakeholders.html.
14. Charon R. The patient-physician relationship. Narrative medicine: a model for empathy, reflection, profession, and trust. *JAMA*. 2001;286(15):1897-1902. Accessed March 10, 2024. https://jamanetwork.com/journals/jama/fullarticle/194300.

Chapter Eleven: How to Share Our Stories in Real Time

1. Frank AW. Not whether but how: considerations on the ethics of telling patients' stories. *Hastings Cent Rep*. 2019;49(6):13-16. Accessed March 12, 2024. https://doi.org/10.1002/hast.1064.
2. O'Brien T. *The Things They Carried*. New York: Houghton Mifflin; 1990. Accessed March 12, 2024. https://dn710001.ca.archive.org/0/items/the-things-they-carried-tim-o-brien/The-Things-They-Carried-Tim-O_Brien.pdf.
3. Ofri D. Doctor-writers: what are the ethics? *Huffington Post*. July 5, 2010. Updated May 25, 2011. Accessed March 12, 2024. https://www.huffpost.com/entry/doctor-writers-what-are-t_b_563664.
4. Rosner, E. The life of Moses Maimonides, a prominent medieval physician. *Einstein Quarterly*. 2002. Accessed March 14, 2024. https://web.archive.org

/web/20090305065423/http://www.aecom.yu.edu/uploadedFiles/EJBM/19Rosner125.pdf.

5. Hirschmann NJ. Gender, Class, and Freedom in Modern Political Theory. Princeton: Princeton University Press; 2009:79.
6. KevinMD. https://www.kevinmd.com/.
7. Silverman E. *The Nocturnists*. Accessed March 14, 2024. https://thenocturnists.org/about.
8. Grumet J. *In My Humble Opinion*. https://jordan-inmyhumbleopinion.blogspot.com/.
9. Grumet J. *The Lives You Touch*. http://www.thelivesyoutouch.com/touchjournal/Publications/Grumet.html.

Chapter Twelve: How Stories Become Reality: Transforming Our Healthcare System

1. Mendoza J. National Health Service (NHS) UK statistics and facts. Statista. December 17, 2025. Accessed March 15, 2024. https://www.statista.com/topics/3128/national-health-service-nhs-uk/#topicOverview.
2. Minhas A. Healthcare expenditure as a share of GDP in the United Kingdom. Statista. March 3, 2026. https://www.statista.com/statistics/317708/healthcare-expenditure-as-a-share-of-gdp-in-the-united-kingdom/.
3. Minhas A. U.S. health expenditure as percent of GDP from 1960 to 2024. Statista. March 3, 2026. https://www.statista.com/statistics/184968/us-health-expenditure-as-percent-of-gdp-since-1960/#:~:text=U.S.%20health%20expenditure%20as%20percent%20of%20GDP%201960%2D2022&text=In%202022%2C%20U.S.%20national%20health,GDP%20share%20among%20developed%20countries.
4. European Observatory on Health Systems and Policies. United Kingdom health system summary 2022. World Health Organization. November 28, 2022. Accessed March 15, 2024. https://eurohealthobservatory.who.int/publications/i/united-kingdom-health-system-summary.
5. Jeffries D, Wellings D, Morris J, Dayan M, Lobont C. Public satisfaction with NHS and social care 2023. The Kings Fund. March 27, 2024. https://www.kingsfund.org.uk/insight-and-analysis/reports/public-satisfaction-nhs-social-care-2023#public-support-principles.
6. Brain J. The birth of the NHS. *Historic UK*. June 30, 2021. Accessed April 2, 2026. https://www.historic-uk.com/HistoryUK/HistoryofBritain/Birth-of-the-NHS/.
7. Moore B, Churchill A. The dawn of the health age. *Nature*. 1911;86:547-549. https://doi.org/10.1038/086547a0.

8. Fischer H. Dr. A.J. Cronin: still persona non grata. *Hektoen International.* Spring 2021. Accessed March 16, 2024. https://hekint.org/2021/06/14/dr-aj-cronin-still-persona-non-grata/.
9. Renowned surgeon and author Dr. Sherwin Nuland shares his story of ECT. Beyond the Body. November 21, 2016. Accessed March 16, 2024. http://www.beyondthebody.org/home/renowned-surgeon-and-author-dr-sherwin-nuland-shares-his-story-of-ect.
10. Newland S. How electroshock therapy changed me. TED YouTube. October 30, 2007. Accessed March 16, 2024. https://www.youtube.com/watch?v=oEZrAGdZ1i8.
11. Davis K. What's to know about electroconvulsive therapy? *MedicalNewsToday.* June 19, 2017. Accessed March 16, 2024. https://www.medicalnewstoday.com/articles/297655#what_is_ECT.
12. Parker J. Study: U.S. ranks 43rd in end-of-life care quality. Hospice News. January 26, 2022. Accessed March 16, 2024. https://hospicenews.com/2022/01/26/study-u-s-ranks-43rd-in-end-of-life-care-quality/.
13. Arapakis K, French E, Jones J. McCauley J. How should we fund end-of-life care in the US? *Lancet Reg Health Am.* 2022;15:100359. Accessed March 16, 2024. https://doi.org/10.1016/j.lana.2022.100359.
14. Riley GF, Lubitz JD. Long-term trends in Medicare payments in the last year of life. *Health Serv Res.* 2010;45(2):565-576. Accessed March 16, 2024. https://doi.org/10.1111/j.1475-6773.2010.01082.x.
15. Gawande A. *Being Mortal.* Metropolitan Books; 2017.
16. Bryant B. Death positive movement fueling hospice growth. *Home Health Care News.* January 7, 2019. Accessed March 16, 2024. https://homehealthcarenews.com/2019/01/death-positive-movement-fueling-hospice-growth/.
17. Dressner MA. Hospital workers: an assessment of occupational injuries and illnesses. Bureau of Labor Statistics Monthly Labor Review. June 2017. Accessed March 17, 2024. https://www.bls.gov/opub/mlr/2017/article/hospital-workers-an-assessment-of-occupational-injuries-and-illnesses.htm.
18. Common injuries among healthcare workers. MultiCare. March 11, 2021. Accessed March 17, 2024. https://www.multicare.org/vitals/common-injuries-among-healthcare-workers/.
19. Preventing violence against health workers. World Health Organization. Accessed March 17, 2024. https://www.who.int/activities/preventing-violence-against-health-workers.
20. 2018 ACEP emergency department violence poll results. American College of Emergency Physicians. September 2018. Accessed March 17, 2024. https://www.emergencyphysicians.org/siteassets/files/pdfs/2018acep-emergency-department-violence-pollresults-2.pdf.